TABLE OF CONTENTS

EXECUTIVE SUMMARY

After consultation with the scientific research community and national organizations that focus on Down syndrome, and taking into account various congressional directives received by the NIH, the NIH Down Syndrome Working Group developed the NIH Research Plan for Down Syndrome. The purpose of the plan is to build upon ongoing NIH-supported research to take advantage of emerging scientific opportunities and set the stage for possible future collaborations in this area.

SELECTED NIH RESEARCH OBJECTIVES

Down Syndrome Research Area	Short-term Objective (0 to 3 Years)	Medium-term Objective (4 to 6 Years)	Long-term Objective (7 to 10 Years)
Pathophysiology of Down Syndrome and Disease Progression	Continue testing cognitive and synaptic function In Down syndrome model mice.	Study whether the impact of aging on certain processes is greater than on others.	Explore genetic and environmental determinants of cognitive function in Down syndrome throughout the lifespan.
Diagnosis, Screening, and Functional Measures	Identify the cognitive phenotype of Down syndrome in a cohort throughout the lifespan.	Link human and mouse cognitive studies relating to Down syndrome.	Develop better measures of hippocampal and cognitive function.
Treatment and Management	Increase research on comorbid psychiatric and medical conditions throughout the lifespan.	Continue learning from the Alzheimer disease research community regarding the best therapeutics.	Investigate the impact of early intervention on psychomotor and cognitive development.
Living with Down Syndrome	Develop a more complete demographic knowledge base.	Study real-world outcomes for Down syndrome families.	Explore new intervention research, especially during transitional stages.
Research Infrastructure	Improve and expand availability of animal models.	Discuss the best mechanisms to use in fostering cross-disciplinary research.	Include cohorts of people with Down syndrome in longitudinal studies.

INTRODUCTION AND BACKGROUND

In early 2006, National Institutes of Health (NIH) Director Dr. Elias Zerhouni asked the National Institute of Child Health and Human Development (NICHD) to take the lead in gathering together program scientists from across the NIH to form a Down Syndrome Working Group. The charge to this group was to coordinate ongoing research already supported by the NIH related to Down syndrome, and to enhance new, NIH-supported research efforts based on identification of areas of greatest scientific opportunity, especially as they relate to the development of future treatments. This plan was developed by the Working Group, with input from the outside scientific and family communities, at the request of Congress in the Labor-HHS-Education Appropriations legislation for fiscal year 2007 (see Appendix B), focusing specifically on genetic and neurobiological research relating to the cognitive dysfunction and the progressive late-life dementia associated with Down syndrome. The purpose of the plan is to build upon ongoing NIH-supported research relating to Down syndrome to reflect the changing lives of individuals and families affected, and to take advantage of emerging scientific opportunities. By organizing the research objectives into groupings according to subject area and timeframes, the plan will also serve to apprise the Down syndrome community of NIH's goals for moving ahead in this area, fostering collaborations between NIH and other agencies and groups.

BACKGROUND ON DOWN SYNDROME
(See also Appendix E)

Named after John Langdon Down, the first physician to describe the syndrome's common features as a distinct entity, Down syndrome is the most frequent genetic cause of mild to moderate mental retardation and associated medical problems. Three genetic variations can cause Down syndrome, which occurs in one out of 800 live births and in all races and economic groups. Most often, Down syndrome is caused by the presence of an extra chromosome 21 in all cells of the individual (called "trisomy 21"). In a small percentage of cases, the extra chromosome 21 is present in some, but not all cells of the individual (called "mosaic trisomy 21"). In about 3 percent to 4 percent of the cases, individuals have the normal number of chromosomes, but carry portions of material from chromosome 21 on other chromosomes, resulting in the features associated with Down syndrome (called "translocation trisomy 21").

A random event during the formation of reproductive cells or during very early development leads to Down syndrome. These events do not appear to be attributable to any behavioral activity of the parents or environmental factors. In almost 9 out of 10 cases, the mother is the source of the extra copy of chromosome 21. As a woman ages, the likelihood that a reproductive cell she ovulates will contain an extra copy of chromosome 21 increases dramatically. A woman younger than age 30 who becomes pregnant has less than a 1 in 1,000 chance of having a baby with Down syndrome, but by age 42, the chance is 1 in 60. However, more than 75 percent of pregnancies that result in Down syndrome occur in women younger than age 40. Several prenatal diagnostic tests are available to detect Down syndrome, including amniocentesis, chorionic villus sampling, and percutaneous umbilical blood sampling.

Physical characteristics of infants born with Down syndrome include epicanthal folds around the eyes, a broad and flat nasal bridge, a round flat face, eyes that slant upwards, small ears, a short neck, and a downward-turned mouth. Medical care for infants born with Down syndrome should include the same well-baby care that other children receive during the first years of life, as well as attention to other health conditions that are more common in children with Down syndrome, including: congenital hypothyroidism, hearing loss, congenital heart disease and pulmonary hypertension, hypotonia (poor muscle tone) and resulting digestive problems, and vision disorders, such as cataracts. During infancy and childhood, children with Down syndrome are 10 to 15 times more likely than other children to develop leukemia, and have a 12-fold higher mortality rate from infectious diseases if the infections are left untreated. However, because more children receive needed medical care, life expectancy for those individuals with Down syndrome has increased dramatically in the United States, from nine years of age in 1959, to 50 years or more today.

Children with Down syndrome may experience developmental delays. However, these children have a wide range of abilities, and each develops at his or her own pace. Many eventually meet developmental milestones. At the other end of the spectrum, adults with Down syndrome age prematurely. Dementia, memory loss, or impaired judgment similar to that occurring in Alzheimer disease patients may appear in adults with Down syndrome. A central focus of ongoing research is to look at Down syndrome across the stages of human development to facilitate effective interventions and treatments.

HIGHLIGHTS OF ONGOING RESEARCH ON DOWN SYNDROME AT THE NIH
(Major research activities, Institutes listed in alphabetical order)

Some of the NIH Institutes and Centers (ICs) have a long-standing history of supporting research relating to Down syndrome. Current research activities of those ICs with significant portfolios in this arena are summarized below.

NATIONAL CANCER INSTITUTE (NCI)

The NCI research program for children with Down syndrome primarily focuses on the acute leukemias that children with Down syndrome are at increased risk for developing. Children with Down syndrome have a cumulative risk for developing leukemia of approximately 2.1 percent by age five years and 2.7 percent by age 30 years. Approximately one-half to two-thirds of the cases of acute leukemia in children with Down syndrome are acute lymphocytic leukemia (ALL). Outcome for Down syndrome children with ALL has generally been reported as poorer than that of non-Down syndrome children, with the lower event-free survival (EFS) and overall survival for children with Down syndrome and ALL appearing to be related to higher rates of treatment-related mortality and to the absence of favorable biological features. Children with Down syndrome and ALL are enrolled on the ALL clinical trials of the NCI-supported

Children's Oncology Group (COG), with the objective of identifying more effective treatments that are adequately tolerated by children with Down syndrome.

Acute myeloid leukemia (AML) in Down syndrome children is biologically and clinically distinctive from AML that occurs in other children. Most children with Down syndrome and AML have the acute megakaryocytic leukemia (AMKL) subtype and have mutations in the *GATA1* gene. The vast majority of cases of AML in children with Down syndrome occur before the age of four years (median age, one year). Infants with Down syndrome also develop transient myeloproliferative disorder (TMD) (also called transient leukemia), a clonal expansion of myeloblasts that can be difficult to distinguish from AML. TMD spontaneously regresses in most cases within the first three months of life, though approximately 20 percent of infants with Down syndrome and TMD eventually develop AML. Down syndrome children with AML have high EFS rates and lower relapse rates compared to non-Down syndrome children with AML. COG clinical trials for children with Down syndrome and AML are focused on reducing the toxicity of treatment while maintaining very high EFS rates and low relapse rates. NCI also supports two investigator-initiated research projects directed toward better understanding the unique biology of AML that occurs in children with Down syndrome.

NATIONAL HEART, LUNG, AND BLOOD INSTITUTE (NHLBI)

The NHLBI funds three projects studying the genetics underlying Down syndrome-related heart malformations, particularly atrioventricular septal defects (AVSD). One project is a human genetics study of Down syndrome patients, with and without ASVDs, to identify gene variants that lead to susceptibility toward heart malformations. The project will subsequently use mouse models to better study how these genes may produce heart defects. Two other projects funded by the NHLBI also use mouse models to study the action of Down syndrome-related genes during the embryonic development of the heart. One is working to characterize the heart malformations in mice that, like trisomy 21 patients, have three copies of many of the genes on human chromosome 21. The other looks specifically at the gene Down Syndrome Critical Region 1 (*Dscr1*) in mouse and chick models of Down syndrome. *Dscr1* is a downstream target of NFATc1 in the developing heart valves. However, restoration of *Dscr1* to disomy did not prevent cardiac or craniofacial abnormalities in trisomic mice, indicating that multiple factors are involved. Current work is underway to analyze the function and interactions of multiple NFATc1 regulatory pathway components in heart valve development. In addition, NHLBI supports numerous grants investigating normal and abnormal valve development. These grants are likely relevant to understanding Down syndrome-related congenital heart defects.

Two other topics relevant to Down syndrome that NHLBI funds are obstructive sleep apnea (OSA) and neurocognitive outcomes of congenital heart disease. The incidence of OSA in Down syndrome children is quite high—greater than 50 percent—and these children likely are susceptible to many of the same outcomes as non-Down syndrome patients with OSA. NHLBI funds several grants investigating the cardiovascular, respiratory, and neurobehavioral consequences of OSA. NHLBI is also funding a randomized controlled study evaluating the efficacy of adenotonsillectomy in OSA patients and investigating potential differences in treatment responses among vulnerable groups, such as overweight children and ethnic minorities.

Children with congenital heart disease show decreased neurocognitive function. However, it is unknown how much of this decreased function is due to cardiovascular insufficiencies caused by the lesions themselves, and how much neural damage results from congenital heart surgery and circulatory arrest. Because a significant percentage of Down syndrome patients require cardiac surgery, and because even a small additional loss of neurocognitive function can have a large impact on quality of life for these patients, methods to reduce risk of neurological damage during surgery are especially important for the Down syndrome population.

Although no studies currently investigate this problem specifically in Down syndrome patients, the NHLBI is funding two studies that compare congenital heart disease surgical patients, who are placed on full circulatory arrest during cardiac surgery or who experience low-flow bypass to controls based on the normative data for the standardized tests they administer. One study follows neurodevelopmental outcomes in patients treated for tetralogy of Fallot, and the other follows patients treated for D-transposition of the great arteries. Investigators will complete both studies in 2009. A third study that NHLBI supports also addresses potential neurological damage during surgery. This study uses a piglet model to evaluate the potential of the drug aprotinin, a serine protease inhibitor, to reduce the risk of brain damage. Genotypic differences may also be a factor in neurocognitive outcomes of congenital heart disease patients. For example, the apolipoprotein E-epsilon2 allele may decrease neuroresiliency when investigators evaluate patients at one year of age. NHLBI currently funds a follow-up study to assess the patients at four years of age.

NATIONAL INSTITUTE ON AGING (NIA)

The NIA has a long-standing interest in Down syndrome and the aging nervous system, cognition, Alzheimer disease, and other neurodegenerative disorders.

Among its research activities are primary intervention studies, including one that tests the use of antioxidants to treat Alzheimer disease in Down syndrome individuals. The objective of this pilot clinical trial is to obtain information on the tolerability, safety, and efficacy of a high potency combinatorial supplement for the treatment of Alzheimer disease in Down syndrome. Individuals with Down syndrome have an increased incidence of Alzheimer disease and evidence of oxidative stress in brain. This double-blind, placebo-controlled trial consists of administration of two cellular antioxidants, and a mitochondrial antioxidant. The investigators are examining the effects on cognition, plasma biomarkers of oxidative stress, beta amyloid levels, and vitamin E levels, in addition to safety/tolerability. The pilot trial should also contribute information as to the possible role of antioxidants in the treatment or prevention of Alzheimer disease in the general population.

Another trial uses vitamin E alone to treat Alzheimer disease in persons with Down syndrome. Persons with Down syndrome are uniquely vulnerable to a form of Alzheimer disease indistinguishable from the sporadic variety that affects aging individuals in the general population. The participants take vitamin E in the form of 1,000 IU capsules, twice daily, for 36 months. This trial evaluates whether high-dose vitamin E will slow the rate of cognitive/functional decline in older individuals with Down syndrome, who are at a very high risk of developing Alzheimer disease.

Individuals with Down syndrome develop the neuropathological hallmarks of Alzheimer disease early in life, and most also experience dementia as they age. Investigators still need to answer a number of key questions about the degenerative process, both in animal models and in the Alzheimer disease and Down syndrome brains. Another study is investigating whether various antioxidant and anti-inflammatory agents used to treat both young and aged mice with partial trisomy (*Ts65Dn*) are effective. NIA also supports research that studies the genes involved in estrogen biosynthesis and estrogen-receptor function and their association with the rate of cognitive decline and risk of Alzheimer disease in women with Down syndrome. This effort aims to identify genetic factors that may modify estrogen levels or estrogen activity and influence risk for Alzheimer disease.

NATIONAL INSTITUTE OF ALLERGY AND INFECTIOUS DISEASES (NIAID)

The NIAID conducts and supports basic and applied research to better understand, treat, and ultimately prevent infectious, immunologic, and allergic diseases. As such, NIAID does not fund research on Down syndrome. NIAID does support basic research on immunology. NIAID-supported researchers recently reported that two genes in the Down syndrome-critical region regulate many genes involved in the development of the immune response. These findings provide a link between the long-established Down syndrome genetic abnormality and the many physical, neurological, and immunological abnormalities observed in these individuals.

Investigators reported that two genes, Down Syndrome Critical Region 1(*DSCR1*) and Dual-specificity Tyrosine-phosphorylation Regulated Kinase 1A (*DYRK1A*), that lie within the Down syndrome-critical region of human chromosome 21 act together to interfere with the nuclear factor of activated T-cells (NFAT) signaling pathway. This pathway is one regulator of vertebrate development. They suggest that the 1.5-fold increase in dosage of *DSCR1* and *DYRK1A* leads to inhibition of NFAT signaling and many of the features of Down syndrome. These predictions are consistent with the researchers' observations of mice that lack components of the NFAT pathway. These mice overexpress the products of the *DSCR1* and *DYRK1A* genes as do mouse models of Down syndrome and humans with trisomy 21. (Arron, et al. [2006]. NFAT dysregulation by increased dosage of *DSCR1* and *DYRK1A* on chromosome 21. *Nature, 441*, 595-600.)

Using genome-wide Ribonucleic Acid (RNA) interference (RNAi) screen in *Drosophila*, other investigators identified regulators of the NFAT signaling pathway. Precise regulation of the NFAT family of transcription factors is essential for vertebrate development and function. The investigators identified a class of proteins as regulators of NFAT signaling. The gene that encodes one of the DYRKs (*DYRK1A*) lies with in the Down syndrome-critical region of human chromosome 21. Overexpression of these negative regulators of NFAT could contribute—by inhibiting NFAT activation—to the neurological and immunological anomalies observed in individuals with trisomy 21. (Gwack, et al. [2006]. A genome-wide *Drosophila* RNAi screen identifies DYRK-family kinases as regulators of NFAT. *Nature, 441*, 646-650.)

NATIONAL INSTITUTE OF CHILD HEALTH AND HUMAN DEVELOPMENT (NICHD)

Since its early years, NICHD has supported a wide range of research related to Down syndrome. These grants include fellowships (F31, F32), career development awards (K08), individual research grants (R01, R03, R21, R37), program project grants (P01), conference grants (R13), and Small Business Innovative Research (SBIR) grants (R43, R44). The studies funded under these various mechanisms include biomedical, behavioral, and biobehavioral studies of different aspects of the complex condition that is Down syndrome.

Some investigations include examination of specific genes or gene clusters and the roles such genes play in the phenotype that is recognized as Down syndrome. Investigators funded by NICHD made seminal contributions to the understanding of the genetics of human chromosome 21 and various mouse chromosomes during the Human Genome Project. Work is ongoing to refine and annotate the genetic maps of both species. Currently, mechanisms by which nondisjunction arises are the focus of two ongoing studies that compare fetal ovarian meiotic events and the impact of ovarian age on the incidence of trisomy. Both genomic and proteomic studies focus on the impact of overexpression of genes located on human chromosome 21 with metabolic pathways in humans with Down syndrome and in mouse models relevant to Down syndrome. These studies include the impact of the trisomic state on mitogen-activated protein (MAP) kinase, calcineurin, and phosphoinositide pathways, mitochondrial function, and on the impact of differential gene expression in various tissues derived from Down syndrome conceptions, including the placenta.

Investigators created and continue to create animal models, typically mice, for studies relevant to cognitive function and dementia in Down syndrome. These include partially trisomic mice, such as *Ts65Dn*, *Ts1Cje*, *Ts2Cje*, and *Ts1Rhr*, as well as partially monosomic mice, such as *Ms1Rhr*. Currently funded studies seek to create mice with partial trisomies of the human chromosome 21 genes located on mouse chromosomes 10 and 17. Investigators who focus on behavioral and biobehavioral studies are designing specific paradigms to assess aspects of cognitive function in animal model systems, such as the effects of overexpression of specific genes in the model organism, *Drosophila,* and determining the location and distribution of specific genes on human chromosome 21 in non-human primates. Electrophysiological studies supported by NICHD of the partially trisomic mice (*Ts65Dn* and *Ts1Cje*) and mice transgenic for specific genes located on human chromosome 21, probe the functional manifestations of the trisomic condition and the impact of specific genes on neuronal function.

NICHD also supports longitudinal studies examining the development and aging of cohorts of individuals who have trisomy of the entire chromosome 21 or partial trisomy to identify genotype/phenotype interactions. One long-standing longitudinal study examines the aging process in individuals with Down syndrome, the incidence of dementia in this population, and factors that impact upon the aging process, including the use of medications such as statins, estrogen replacement therapy, and specific antioxidants. Another effort is following a cohort of partially trisomic individuals and designing specific animal model systems to investigate aspects of the genotype/phenotype relationship.

In addition, several behavioral and biobehavioral studies utilize Down syndrome individuals as "control" groups for determining similarities and differences associated with Williams syndrome, Fragile X syndrome, Rett syndrome, Prader Willi syndrome, or idiopathic mental retardation. One grantee is studying unique aspects of developmental trajectories and is designing new tests to elucidate similarities and differences associated with intellectual disability, including Down syndrome. Several NICHD-funded investigators are focusing their research on family events and dynamics, and on whether family influences on social outcome, family adaptation to dual diagnosis, and sibling interactions during infancy. One NICHD program project grant focuses on facilitating communication among individuals with severe intellectual disability, including individuals with Down syndrome.

A recent clinical trial funded by NICHD conducted extensive prenatal screening to determine the best combination of diagnostic procedures. Another trial is testing the impact of vitamin E therapy in adults with Down syndrome older than age 50 years.

Among the small business initiatives supported by NICHD, one focuses on diagnostic proteomic profiles for aneuploidy, and another project focuses on weight-loss programs for adults with intellectual disabilities. Still other researchers have developed computer-assisted learning strategies for children with intellectual disabilities, including individuals with Down syndrome, and have designed handheld assistive devices to facilitate time management and scheduling.

In addition, investigators in the NICHD Division of Intramural Research are conducting a study to evaluate the potential of growth factors to prevent or reduce the intellectual disability associated with Down syndrome in a mouse model. These investigators previously showed that, because of its critical role in embryonic growth and development, a peptide (vasoactive intestinal peptide) protects against oxidative stress and ameliorates learning deficits in a model of fetal alcohol syndrome.

Several recent conference grants supported in part by NICHD include meetings at which participants discussed the biology of human chromosome 21 genes and cognition and behavior in Down syndrome. The NICHD also has provided partial support for several of the biennial international meetings of Down syndrome investigators. Recently, NICHD convened a meeting of experts to hear their recommendations for future research directions.

NATIONAL INSTITUTE OF MENTAL HEALTH (NIMH)

NIMH's research interests include investigations that attempt to assess the rates of comorbid mental illnesses in Down syndrome, including, for example, autism, pervasive developmental disorder, obsessive-compulsive disorder, depression, and psychosis, as well as studies of behavioral or psychopharmacological interventions for comorbid disorders within this population.

Specifically, NIMH has an active program announcement, *Research on Psychopathology in Intellectual Disabilities*. This announcement is designed to support research on comorbid mental disorders within the intellectually disabled population, including individuals with Down syndrome. Some examples of projects that NIMH is currently supporting from this announcement include: 1) an international longitudinal study of the course and pattern of psychopathology, and biopsychosocial risk and protective factors associated with psychopathology, in children with intellectual disabilities, including children with Down syndrome; and 2) a large study of the impact of stress on functioning, and coping strategies utilized to reduce stress, in adults with intellectual disabilities, including those with Down syndrome.

Individuals with Down syndrome have deficits in fine motor learning and have a disproportionately small cerebellum, a brain region that plays an important role in movement. To identify genes that may contribute to these deficits, intramural researchers at NIMH are using mouse models of Down syndrome to investigate how extra copies of certain genes impact specific cell types in the cerebellum.

NATIONAL INSTITUTE OF NEUROLOGICAL DISORDERS AND STROKE (NINDS)

The NINDS currently funds basic, clinical, and translational research on a broad range of disorders affecting the brain, spinal cord, and nerves of the body, including research on or related to Down syndrome.

One funded project aims to clarify the role of a protein called amyloid precursor protein (APP) in neuronal degeneration in a mouse model of Down syndrome. The gene for APP is located on human chromosome 21 and is present in three copies in Down syndrome and its mouse models. Abnormal processing of APP is implicated in Alzheimer disease, which can develop in Down syndrome patients as early as middle age. The investigators in this study will determine whether and, if so, how excess APP disrupts the function of a neuronal growth factor important for neuronal survival. Another protein whose gene maps to the Down syndrome-associated region of human chromosome 21 is Down syndrome cell-adhesion molecule (DSCAM). Although the role of DSCAM in the neurological characteristics of Down syndrome is not yet clear, understanding its functions in experimental models may provide insights into the causes and consequences of developmental abnormalities in the human disease. In the fruit fly *Drosophila*, the homologous protein Dscam guides early stages of neuronal circuit development, and a study supported by NINDS will focus on how different forms of Dscam function in establishing specific neuronal connections. The expression levels of many other proteins are also affected by the extra genetic material from chromosome 21 in Down syndrome, and another NINDS-supported study will compare global protein-expression levels in normal mice and Down syndrome model mice. Identifying these changes in protein expression will allow further research into how they contribute to disease phenotypes.

In addition to these studies on Down syndrome or Down syndrome-related proteins, other research in the NINDS portfolio is also relevant to understanding this disease and its consequences for nervous system development and function throughout life. For example, research into the structure and function of neurons and neuronal circuits advances the understanding of how abnormalities, such as those seen in Down syndrome, can lead to cognitive deficits. In February 2005, NINDS held a workshop entitled *Down Syndrome: Toward Optimal Synaptic Function and Cognition*. The goals of this workshop were to review recent advances in Down syndrome research and relevant technical approaches, and to identify key priority areas for future work, including a focus on developing ways to improve cognitive function. The workshop recommendations are described in a published report (see Appendix C).

RESEARCH AREAS AND OBJECTIVES

Initially formed in late 2005, the NIH Down Syndrome Working Group first met to share the research activities related to Down syndrome that the NIH was supporting, and to discuss how the NIH Institutes and Centers could better coordinate their efforts and share their specific expertise. After consultation with the biomedical and behavioral scientific and research advocacy communities, and considering other information largely gathered through a series of facilitated, targeted meetings (see Appendix C), the Working Group developed the following list of research priorities to complement and guide its future efforts regarding Down syndrome. The objectives are listed according to research themes and are further grouped by the estimated, but realistic, timeframe that it could take to accomplish them. For the purposes of this document, "short-term" is defined as beginning from the date of publication of this document through approximately three years from that time, "medium-term" is approximately four to six years from that time, and "long-term" runs from seven to 10 years or beyond.

PATHOPHYSIOLOGY OF DOWN SYNDROME AND DISEASE PROGRESSION

Investigators mapped the first two of several hundred genes mapped to human chromosome 21 in 1973. By 2000, a consortium of investigators published the Deoxyribonucleic Acid (DNA) sequence of chromosome 21. Once the genes on chromosome 21 were identified, it was possible to identify the effects of having an extra copy of individual genes or clusters of genes. To study these effects, researchers use animal model systems, including fully or partially trisomic mice, which have features of the human prototype not seen in other animal models.

Short-term Objectives
1. Continue **testing cognitive and synaptic function** in Down syndrome model mice focusing specifically on relevant genes located on human chromosome 21.

2. **Develop mouse models to study synaptic and vesicular trafficking** (these may exist, but may not be utilized for Down syndrome research at the current time). Allow studies of other disorders associated with intellectual and developmental disabilities (Fragile X, Rett syndrome, etc.) to guide and inform directions for such studies.

3. **Expand and improve proteomic, metabolomic, transcriptomics, and phenomic approaches**, including:

- Appropriate sample preparation techniques to create suitable proteomic samples from mouse brains;
- Fractionation techniques to visualize the perhaps 100,000 proteins that exist;
- Additional proteomic methods beyond two-dimensional gels;
- Rigorous statistical techniques to determine whether a statistically significant change in protein levels has biologic relevance;
- Methods to relate findings in the mouse to humans;
- Research beyond proteins and proteomics, using emerging techniques to move into metabolites and metabolomics, and begin to examine what generates alterations in learning and memory; and
- Linking data from transcripts to the proteome, metabolome, and phenome.

4. Study **pathways and cascades** affected in Down syndrome. These might include pathways that affect mitochondrial function (adenosine triphosphate [ATP] production), calcineurin, MAP kinases, and oxidative stress. Link up with relevant research into specific gene effects at other Institutes, and explore the effects on modulation of development in other organ systems.

Medium-term Objectives

1. Study whether the **impact of aging on physiologic and cognitive processes** is greater than on others. Such research probably requires a range of longitudinal studies of more than five years' duration, with different emphases. For example, studies could include:

   - The non-demented population with Down syndrome, which is likely to be heterogeneous and may include people in the early stages of unrecognized Alzheimer disease.
   - Understanding the factors that affect the risk of dementia, and what factors may be associated with not developing dementia. Some people with Down syndrome do not develop dementia by their late 60s or early 70s. To complete such studies, researchers would also need to better understand the clinical course of dementia in people with Down syndrome.
   - Consider research with different subpopulations of individuals with Down syndrome to examine variations in aging patterns. Much literature focuses on early development and on individuals older than age 40, but very little research targets people with Down syndrome during their 20s and 30s.

2. Sequence the **developmental events of abnormal spine development**, including genetics and cellular aspects (this research may interface with a common theme in developmental disabilities and could include information from other disorders, such as Fragile X and Rett syndromes).

3. Study the biochemistry of **APP processing** in humans with Down syndrome and in animal models (including mechanisms of trafficking and Abeta production, degradation, and clearance).

4. Describe more fully the **mitochondrial dysfunction** in Down syndrome and the exact status of mitochondrial function; develop targeted therapies for mitochondrial function in Down syndrome.

   - Assess endocytosis and endosomal trafficking *in vivo* and *in vitro*.
   - Assess failed signaling and related neurotrophic deficits to help determine the relationship between disease progression and cognitive deficits.

5. Study **synaptic vesicle trafficking** in Down syndrome and postsynaptic mechanisms including metabotropic and ionotropic glutamate receptors and other neurotransmitter receptors.

6. Develop a strategy to **correlate descriptive studies** of human and Down syndrome model mouse development over the lifespan. This strategy will inform the development of a cognitive phenotype for Down syndrome that will support longitudinal studies (see below).

Long-term Objectives

1. Explore **genetic and environmental determinants** of cognitive function in Down syndrome throughout the lifespan. This work may involve long-term (more than 10 years) study of existing and new cohorts of individuals.

2. Connect **cellular mechanisms** and genotype to synaptic and cognitive phenotype.

DIAGNOSIS, SCREENING, AND FUNCTIONAL MEASURES

The science of assessment has evolved in recent years, and while significantly more options for diagnostic and screening measures are now available, it will be important for researchers to capitalize on these advances in measurement. For example, utilization of more specialized measures of functioning across domains would allow more fine-grained analysis and phenotyping, which may assist in identification of biomarkers.

To proceed, the scientific community needs to focus on improving their tools, techniques, methods and measures, moving toward a minimum set of common measures for use across studies, age groups, and developmental and behavioral domains. In addition, the field may benefit from an agreement on common domains to be assessed for clinical research in Down syndrome (e.g. non-verbal problem-solving ability, language and communication skills, adaptive functioning), to allow for comparability across studies, noting that those appropriate for one stage of life may not be appropriate for others.

Short-term Objectives

1. **Identify the cognitive phenotype of Down syndrome** in a cohort throughout the lifespan, and link the phenotype to cognitive defects and developmental standards. This could include defining speech and language, behavioral, and psychological abnormalities, using magnetic resonance imaging (MRI) and functional MRI (fMRI) to examine major pathways and determining how those pathways differ in persons with Down syndrome.

2. In addition, researchers need to apply standardized instruments and criteria to **define the clinical profile of Alzheimer disease in Down syndrome**; these instruments must be sensitive to the baseline-level function of this population. Standardizing a cognitive battery in mice to help develop a core set of measures for this purpose would help researchers.

3. **Collect and bank well-characterized organs for postmortem research**. Such specimens are necessary for understanding the factors that underlie dementia in people with Down syndrome. Increasing banking of organs from individuals with Down syndrome who were older than age 40 years at the time of death would help to identify the brain correlates of clinical signs and symptoms.

4. Expand the **brain imaging project** supported by the Foundation for the NIH. This project has enrolled 400 people and might expand to include an adequate sample of people with Down syndrome. Undertake a systematic **analysis of the development of key structures in the brains** of people with Down syndrome at various developmental stages using standardized techniques and measurements. Imaging studies of normal development currently in progress and supported by the NIH could inform this endeavor.

5. **Develop new statistical approaches**. Data from partial trisomy patients can generate vectors of pathways and ways to constrain them.

6. Consider developing **additional outcome measures for use in clinical trials** to offer supplementary options for assessing change across domains of functioning.

Medium-term Objectives

1. **Link human and mouse cognitive studies** relating to Down syndrome to:

   - Better characterize cognitive deficits in mice from the psychological/psychiatric/functional aspects;
   - Develop standardized methods to test synaptic and cognitive function in Down syndrome model mice; and
   - Develop tests that "tap" into the same "cognitive" processes in both mice and humans (such as discriminative taste aversion).

2. Establish whether and how **synaptic dysfunction correlates to abnormal cognition**, and determine the best phenotype/genotype markers for therapeutic screening.

3. Develop **nanotechnology approaches** to enhance contrast of imaging reagents for finer resolution studies in younger populations with Down syndrome.

4. Explore whether **magnetic resonance spectroscopy**, which can show changes much earlier than neurocognitive exams, offers another promising technology for studying neuron health in individuals with Down syndrome.

5. **Assay specific vulnerable brain regions**, such as the hippocampus, cerebellum, and prefrontal cortex, from a prospective developmental perspective using standard measures and techniques, enhancing current cognitive batteries applicable at specific stages across the lifespan.

Long-term Objectives

1. Develop better **measures of hippocampal and cognitive function** in persons with Down syndrome.

TREATMENT AND MANAGEMENT

For individuals with Down syndrome and their families, there is a continuing need to study clinical treatments and interventions. Moreover, at least half of all children with Down syndrome have a comorbid condition. Two conditions that have the potential to have significant impact on cognitive function during the first few years of life are the development of leukemia and the high incidence of congenital heart disease. Both of these conditions necessitate extensive medical intervention.

Short-term Objectives

1. **Expand research on comorbid psychiatric and medical conditions** that occur throughout the lifespan, including depression, dementia, and various developmental disabilities. Other comorbid conditions that could benefit from concerted interdisciplinary efforts include the following:

   - *Leukemias*—Early medical or behavioral interventions can alter the developmental trajectory in children treated for leukemias. These children have concomitant behavioral and cognitive difficulties; for example, 40 percent had an Intelligence Quotient (IQ) of less than 75 on follow-up one to three years after treatment. The extent of problems typically depends on the age of the child at treatment, its intensity, and the time lapsed since treatment. Children with an underlying trisomic disorder that affects the brain's development who undergo this intensive treatment for leukemia are likely to face problems for at least several years. Future research could build on studies such as a new clinical trial of methotrexate and neurocognitive outcomes that may provide information on the mechanisms by which impairments occur.
   - *Congenital heart disease*—As survival of children with congenital heart defects improves, clinicians increasingly recognize neurodevelopmental problems in at least half of survivors. The incidence of neurodevelopmental problems seems to increase over time. Children with congenital heart disease have a fairly characteristic neurodevelopmental signature. As adolescents, they tend to have difficulty with social

cognition. However, the impact on children with Down syndrome is less clear. Neurodevelopmental outcomes vary, even in children who have the same defects and receive the same treatments and may be related to specific allelic variants of genes not located on human chromosome 21. Children with Down syndrome who are treated for heart defects probably have worse neurodevelopmental outcomes than children without Down syndrome. Possible research opportunities could include longitudinal assessments of cognitive and behavioral outcomes in relation to genetic studies.

- *Obstructive sleep apnea (OSA)*—As with typically developing individuals, this condition may exert an impact on cognition in individuals with Down syndrome.
- Other comorbid conditions that deserve more thorough investigation in Down syndrome individuals throughout the lifespan include:
  - *Seizure disorders*
  - *Psychiatric or neurobehavioral problems*
  - *Celiac disease*
  - *Atlanto-axial instability*
  - *Endocrine function*

2. Review earlier literature on **understanding and improving the motor skills** of individuals with Down syndrome, with particular attention to whether and how sensory structures in persons with Down syndrome are altered. In addition, review current relevant NIH-supported research that is not specific to Down syndrome, but may be applicable.

3. Determine whether individuals with cognitive impairment, including those with Down syndrome, could be considered as candidates for **transplantation studies**.

4. Review findings from current **clinical trials of vitamin E and antioxidants** in individuals with Alzheimer disease, and determine whether to test these substances in persons with Down syndrome to see if they might enhance the function of circuits involved in cognition.

5. **Test drugs** used by persons with Alzheimer disease in mouse models of Down syndrome, and eventually in other model systems, to determine their effects on cognition.

6. Encourage **testing of "orphan drugs"** in animal and cellular models to determine potential beneficial effects on cognition in individuals with Down syndrome.

Medium-term Objectives

In general, one challenge faced by researchers is how to focus on precisely targeting time windows for early therapeutics, in relation to the use of available treatments for individuals with Down syndrome, as well as the development of new agents.

1. Continue the dialog with the Alzheimer disease research community regarding the best **anti-amyloids and other agents' use as early therapeutics**.

2. Encourage studies to understand the best **use of therapeutics over time** in a Down syndrome population. For instance, few researchers have described studies of adults with Down

syndrome treated with **Aricept®**. Because the progression of cognitive decline in different stages of dementia is not linear, this medication is likely to have differential efficacy depending on when in the pathological cascade it is used.

3. Explore the impact of cholesterol on dementia. People who have Down syndrome and **cholesterol levels** higher than 200 mg/dl are at substantially higher risk for dementia than people with lower cholesterol levels. However, the risk of dementia in people with high cholesterol who take **statins** is the same as in people with lower cholesterol levels.

4. Explore the specific impact of **hormone replacement therapy (HRT)** use on women with Down syndrome. Women with Down syndrome experience **menopause** at an earlier age and are at increased risk for dementia compared to women who are older at onset of menopause. Some studies show that taking HRT appears to protect episodic memory tasks in women who did not have dementia at baseline. In addition, women who took HRT had better scores on one cognitive measure over a 14- to 18-month period, but HRT had no effect on any of the other measures. Currently, the data are not sufficient to show whether HRT reduces the cumulative risk for Alzheimer disease.

5. Consider developing funding opportunities for **translational research** that applies findings from literature review **on motor skills** in individuals with Down syndrome.

6. Further investigate the **resting state hypothesis** to assess default activity. Data suggest that the resting state differs in those with Alzheimer disease or mild cognitive impairment.

Long-term Objectives

Children with Down syndrome have greater deficits in auditory short-term memory than children with equivalent IQs. Researchers examining whether these deficits influence the benefits of language intervention for children with Down syndrome may be warranted, and may lead to more refinement of behavioral interventions for speech and language development.

1. Investigate the impact of **early intervention or infant stimulation** on the psychomotor and cognitive development of Down syndrome children.

2. Identify **compensatory strategies**. Children with Down syndrome need therapies that help them process available linguistic input, matching individual differences in children with Down syndrome to those therapies best suited to their profiles.

3. Develop **cross-disciplinary collaborations** (e.g., educational psychologists, psychiatrists, neurophysiologists) **and public-private partnerships** to test educational, pharmaceutical, and therapeutic interventions. Investigators should take ethical considerations into account when testing any interventions in individuals with Down syndrome.

LIVING WITH DOWN SYNDROME

Studies of family and classroom environments may provide information that allows us to maximize biobehavioral interventions for improving daily-life function and cognition of people with Down syndrome.

Short-term Objectives

1. Develop a more complete **demographic** knowledge base of individuals with Down syndrome and their families. Surprisingly little is known about the demographics of families with a child who has Down syndrome, except that these children are more likely to have older mothers. One in eight mothers of children with Down syndrome is aged 40 years or older, compared to 1.8 percent of mothers of other children. Older mothers likely are better educated than younger mothers. The mothers of children with Down syndrome are also more likely to be white.

2. Develop a **Web page containing information on Down syndrome** and related research, similar to the condition-specific NIH Web pages for autism or other disorders. The page should include user-friendly information relevant to both the research and family communities. This page should also include links to information about pending clinical trials and diagnosis and treatment guidelines adopted by nationally recognized professional societies. (The Alzheimer Disease Education Referral site managed by the NIA may be a possible model.)

3. Examine closely the **impact of Down syndrome on families and schools**. Possible research questions include how families react to children with Down syndrome, who may have fewer maladaptive behaviors than children with other disabilities, but they do have some of the behaviors. Many families of a child with Down syndrome want integrated schooling, but there is little comparative research on whether it has beneficial effects, and many families also worry about what will happen to their children once they leave the school system.

Medium-term Objectives

1. As children with Down syndrome live longer, study **real-world outcomes** for the family. These topics include the health of the family, the lifespan of parents, sibling educational attainment, and when siblings marry and have children. Such work could include:

   - Identifying the factors that lead to positive and negative outcomes in families that have an individual member with Down syndrome.
   - Conducting research on the intergenerational transmission of caregiving responsibilities and how best to foster those transitions.

2. Research and develop and/or adapt **assistive devices** that facilitate integration into society.

Long-term Objectives

1. Explore **new intervention research** in families, schools, and residential environments that integrates the transition from late adolescence to young adulthood, as well as ways to enhance physical fitness. Such research results could be disseminated for use by other agency programs and in community settings.

RESEARCH INFRASTRUCTURE

Short-term Objectives

1. Improve and expand availability of **animal models** for research on Down syndrome. Distribution of mouse models remains a chronic problem. Although some researchers distribute their models freely, the number of researchers who wish to use them has tripled, yet supplies of the animals are limited, the animals are expensive to purchase, and they require complex husbandry. As a result, investigators cannot afford to obtain enough of these mice for their research. Researchers need the available animal models to be inexpensive and made available as early in their development as possible. Researchers also need a central facility with several dissemination sites. However, investigators need to share the models they develop while they maintain their ability to publish their findings in high-quality journals. To achieve these goals, it would be necessary to:

   - Explore improvements to the *Tc1* model. One strategy might be to attach an intact human chromosome 21 to a mouse chromosome, which should result in more stable retention of the human chromosome, making the model much more powerful.
   - Establish a mouse "core" to create the models needed for today's research and to also predict what mouse strains and reagents researchers are likely to need in the near future. The cores could be useful for moving from genotype to phenotype and for helping to determine the involvement of a specific gene in specific phenotypes. Increase the number of animal models and make them available (currently under a contract mechanism).
   - Find ways to reduce the cost of animal models to NIH-funded investigators.

2. Develop **other new model systems** and improve existing models, such as:

   - Develop new model systems at organismal and cellular level to study aspects of Down syndrome.
   - Add other organs (in addition to brains) as model systems.
   - Deploy studies in additional organisms such as *C. elegans* and *Drosophila* that involve perturbation of individual chromosome 21 genes, and study the effects on the differentiation and maturation of individual neurons and synapses.

3. Develop a **coherent program of analysis**. The genetic heritage of people with Down syndrome has a great deal to teach about the health of everyone. Researchers should be encouraged to analyze genetic modifiers to show how they contribute to the many phenotypes in Down syndrome and the rest of the population. Once researchers identify a region of chromosome 21 for further study and a mouse model is available, they can ask similar questions when using single-gene models.

Medium-term Objectives

1. Convene a meeting of the NIH leadership (or their representatives) from the Institutes and Centers involved in the NIH Down Syndrome Working Group to discuss the **best mechanisms to use** in fostering cross-disciplinary, collaborative, and clinical research on Down syndrome, in addition to the work already being supported. To inform this discussion, the Working Group should review ongoing international collaborative efforts relating to research on Down syndrome. Further, the Working Group should follow up with more specific discussions about cost, duplication, infrastructure, and training; whether to focus on basic, translational, or clinical research; and what specific avenues of inquiry to follow.

2. Consider ways to **include participants with Down syndrome** in NIH-funded clinical trials. NIH should review existing infrastructure, such as the Clinical and Translational Science Awards or the National Children's Study, for possible inclusion of this population. NIH program scientists who write Funding Opportunity Announcements could also consider including, where relevant, individuals with Down syndrome. Some examples of possible opportunities for research studies involving individuals with Down syndrome are:

   - The impact of novel medications on cognitive enhancement, daily function, or behavioral disorders.
   - Appropriate interventions for congenital heart disease and obstructive sleep apnea.
   - Therapies used for individuals with Alzheimer disease.

3. To enhance enrollment of individuals with Down syndrome, consider using **telemedicine** to screen and enroll subjects at distant sites. (Completion of a feasibility study using telemedicine to diagnose dementia in Down syndrome enabled researchers to obtain funding to continue testing the reliability of this method.)

4. Establish a centralized **brain, cell, tissue, DNA, RNA bank**; correlate the nature and severity of cognitive deficits and age of onset and severity of dementia. (Currently, the NICHD maintains a multi-disease bank of brain and other tissue that has some Down syndrome fetal material, but the demand for tissues far outweighs availability. The major challenges are to obtain permission to collect samples and to obtain tissue prepared appropriately.)

5. Support **database development**. Determine what databases currently exist (including those already developed for other conditions, and in development internationally), and whether potential collaborations might be feasible; involve National Library of Medicine in the development of any new databases.

6. Establish or expand **training programs for clinician/scientists** in research relevant to Down syndrome. Such training is critical for moving any research plan for Down syndrome into the future.

7. Assist researchers in assembling **demographically representative samples**, to better allow scientists to determine which findings they can generalize to a larger population of people with Down syndrome in the United States, especially across their lifespans.

8. **Establish a regular collaboration** between the NIH and the larger community of parent groups and researchers. The NIH Down Syndrome Working Group should continue to meet periodically with outside groups to share progress on research and hear about pressing concerns facing families. These meetings could help the community better understand how Down syndrome research is supported across the NIH. These meetings could also serve as a sounding board for current research issues, such as the best ways to recruit participants, and to better understand the evolving needs of families and individuals with Down syndrome.

9. Support a scientific meeting to highlight and assess **best practices in the use of tests** clinical researchers currently use at different developmental stages.

Long-term Objectives

1. Continue to include cohorts of people with Down syndrome in appropriate **longitudinal and cross-sectional studies**, e.g. a longitudinal cohort study of children with Down syndrome with and without congenital heart disease. Investigators could study the cohort *in utero* and follow-up using structural and neural imaging.

2. To ensure applicability of research findings to all segments of the population, **expand outreach efforts to recruit** individuals who have Down syndrome and who are members of racial and ethnic minorities for clinical trials. (Lack of a diverse sample of research participants has hampered research efforts. In part, this dearth may occur because Caucasian people with Down syndrome live until their 50s and 60s, but those of other races die younger. In addition, although some parents are hesitant to involve their children in longitudinal clinical trials, others are eager to participate in research, in part, because the types of information and resources offered to parents vary widely across the United States.)

IMPLEMENTATION OF RESEARCH OBJECTIVES

This plan, *The NIH Research Plan for Down Syndrome*, was developed by the NIH Down Syndrome Working Group with a significant amount of input from the scientific community outside of the NIH, as well as key organizations that represent researchers involved in this area and individuals with Down syndrome and their families. The research plan is intended to provide the NIH, and its member Institutes and Centers, with guidelines for prioritizing and coordinating future research related to Down syndrome, whether basic, translational, or clinical, and whether funded by one Institute or several. The plan will also help to communicate NIH's priorities for research related to Down syndrome to the wider scientific community, hopefully encouraging the submission of a new slate of investigator-initiated applications. As funding permits, the NIH Down Syndrome Working Group intends to work cooperatively on new Funding Opportunity Announcements that will begin to implement the research objectives described in the plan.

Many individuals with Down syndrome are living longer and becoming more integrated into schools and the workforce. Consequently, the research related to new health issues, including those related to cognition and learning, needs to be addressed by a wider range of federal agencies and programs, making coordination both more challenging and more appropriate. At the same time, the clear need for research and programs for people with Down syndrome and their families, and the limitations on human and fiscal resources, require that each agency focus on its particular types of expertise without unnecessary duplication. The NIH Down Syndrome Working Group hopes to serve in a coordinating role for the NIH in working with other agencies and the patient/family advocacy organizations, possibly collaborating with them on future research endeavors.

APPENDIX A: NIH DOWN SYNDROME WORKING GROUP MEMBERS

NATIONAL INSTITUTE OF CHILD HEALTH AND HUMAN DEVELOPMENT (NICHD)
Mary Lou Oster-Granite, Ph.D. (Chair)
Yvonne Maddox, Ph.D.
Lisa Kaeser, J.D.
Dana Bynum

NATIONAL INSTITUTE OF NEUROLOGICAL DISORDERS AND STROKE (NINDS)
Robert Riddle, Ph.D.
Heather Rieff, Ph.D.
Cara Allen, Ph.D.

NATIONAL INSTITUTE ON AGING (NIA)
Laurie Ryan, Ph.D.
Kathie Reed

NATIONAL INSTITUTE OF MENTAL HEALTH (NIMH)
Lisa Gilotty, Ph.D.
Alison Bennett

NATIONAL HEART, LUNG, AND BLOOD INSTITUTE (NHLBI)
Charlene Schramm, Ph.D.
Stephanie Burrows

NATIONAL INSTITUTE ON DEAFNESS AND OTHER COMMUNICATION DISORDERS (NIDCD)
Judith Cooper, Ph.D.
Buck Wong

NATIONAL CANCER INSTITUTE (NCI)
Malcolm Smith, M.D., Ph.D.
Susan Erickson

NATIONAL INSTITUTE OF ALLERGY AND INFECTIOUS DISEASES (NIAID)
Josiah Wedgwood, Ph.D.
Francesca Maccharini, Ph.D.
Jill Harper

NATIONAL INSTITUTE OF DENTAL AND CRANIOFACIAL RESEARCH (NIDCR)
Rochelle Small, Ph.D.
Isabel Garcia

NATIONAL INSTITUTE ON DRUG ABUSE (NIDA)
Larry Stanford, Ph.D.
Geoffrey Laredo

OFFICE OF THE NIH DIRECTOR, OFFICE OF RESEARCH SERVICES (NIH/OD/ORS)
Diane Cooper, M.S.L.S., A.H.I.P.

APPENDIX B: CONGRESSIONAL DIRECTIVES, FISCAL YEAR 2007

The House and Senate Appropriations Committees, in their committee reports for Labor-HHS-Education for fiscal year 2007, included the following language on Down syndrome in the NIH portions of the reports.

HOUSE (REPT. 109-515)

Office of the NIH Director

Down Syndrome—The Committee encourages the Director to establish an NIH Down syndrome research task force on cognition to develop a strategic plan for genetic and neurobiological research relating to the cognitive dysfunction and the progressive late-life dementia associated with Down syndrome. The purpose of the strategic plan is to provide a guide for coordinating Down syndrome research on cognition across NIH and for enhancing the development of new research efforts based on identification of areas of greatest scientific opportunity, especially as they relate to the development of future treatments. The plan should include short, intermediate and long-term goals for basic and clinical research with strategies for achieving goals and with specified time frames for implementation.

NINDS

Down Syndrome—As a follow-up to its successful Down syndrome workshop to address research priorities relating to the synaptic structure and function of neuronal circuits, NINDS is encouraged to issue program announcements related to its workshop findings. Specifically, the Committee encourages NINDS to support investigations relating to the genetic and cellular basis for abnormalities in the structure and function of neuronal circuits in both developing and mature nervous systems. NINDS is also encouraged to work with the Office of the Director, OPASI [Office of Portfolio Analysis and Strategic Initiatives], and other Institutes to develop a strategic plan for Down syndrome research and to coordinate all Down syndrome research within NIH. In anticipation of future clinical trials that will seek to measure accurately cognitive improvement in individuals with Down syndrome, the Committee further encourages NINDS to develop better measurement standards and a common data base that can be used generally for such trials.

NICHD

Down Syndrome—NICHD is encouraged to partner with NINDS and other agencies to define additional mouse models needed to link important structural and functional abnormalities that underlie cognitive difficulties to the actions of specific genes and gene pathways.

NIA

Down Syndrome—The Committee commends NIA for its support of studies to examine the cellular, molecular, and genetic bases for age-related neuropathological and cognitive abnormalities in people with Down syndrome. The Committee encourages NIA to further examine these abnormalities and to devise new methods for diagnosing and treating them. Given that all people with Down syndrome develop the neuropathological changes of Alzheimer disease, and that many or most go on to suffer dementia, NIA is further encouraged to consider how studies of the Down syndrome population might enhance the ability to understand, diagnose and treat Alzheimer disease.

NIMH

Down Syndrome—The Committee encourages NIMH to develop new strategies for cataloging, understanding, diagnosing, and treating behavioral disorders that are common in people with Down syndrome, including autism, pervasive developmental disorder, obsessive compulsive disorder, depression, and psychosis. The Committee encourages NIMH to coordinate its research on Down syndrome with NICHD, NINDS, NIA, and other Institutes.

SENATE (REPT. 109-287)

Office of the NIH Director

Down Syndrome—The Committee urges the Director of NIH to establish an NIH Down syndrome research task force on cognition to develop a strategic plan for genetic and neurobiological research relating to the cognitive dysfunction and the progressive late-life dementia associated with Down syndrome. The purpose of the strategic plan is to provide a guide for coordinating Down syndrome research on cognition across NIH and for enhancing the development of new research efforts based on identification of areas of greatest scientific opportunity, especially as they relate to the development of future treatments. The plan should include short-, intermediate- and long-term goals for basic and clinical research with strategies for achieving goals and with specified time frames for implementation.

NINDS

Down Syndrome—As a follow-up to its successful Down syndrome workshop to address research priorities relating to the synaptic structure and function of neuronal circuits, NINDS is strongly encouraged to issue special program announcements related to its workshop findings. Specifically, the Committee encourages NINDS to identify and fund investigations relating to the genetic and cellular basis for abnormalities in the structure and function of neuronal circuits in both the developing and mature nervous systems. NINDS is also encouraged to work with the Office of the Director, OPASI, and the other Institutes to develop a strategic plan for Down syndrome research and to coordinate all Down syndrome research within NIH. In anticipation of future clinical trials that will seek to accurately measure cognitive improvement in individuals with Down syndrome, the Committee further encourages NINDS to begin to develop better measurement standards and a common database that can be used generally for such trials.

NICHD

Down Syndrome—NICHD is encouraged to partner with NINDS and other agencies to define additional mouse models needed to link important structural and functional abnormalities that underlie cognitive difficulties to the actions of specific genes and gene pathways. The Committee also encourages NICHD to work with the Office of the Director, OPASI, and the other Institutes to develop a strategic plan for Down syndrome research and to coordinate its research within NIH.

NIA

Down Syndrome—The Committee commends NIA for its support of studies to examine the cellular, molecular, and genetic bases for age-related neuropathological and cognitive abnormalities in people with Down syndrome. It encourages NIA to further examine these abnormalities and to devise new methods for diagnosing and treating them. Given that all people with Down syndrome develop the neuropathological changes of Alzheimer disease, and that many or most go on to suffer dementia, NIA is encouraged to consider how studies of the Down syndrome population might enhance the ability to understand, diagnose and treat Alzheimer disease. The Committee encourages NIA to coordinate its research with NICHD, NINDS, NIMH, and other Institutes.

NIMH

Down Syndrome—The Committee encourages NIMH to develop new strategies for cataloging, understanding, diagnosing, and treating behavioral disorders that are common in people with Down syndrome. They include autism, pervasive developmental disorder, obsessive compulsive disorder, depression, and psychosis. The Committee urges NIMH to coordinate its research on Down syndrome with NICHD, NINDS, NIA, and other Institutes.

APPENDIX C: MEETINGS AND CONSULTATIONS

The NIH Down Syndrome Working Group considered (but did not necessarily adopt) information from and suggestions made during the following meetings and consultations in drafting this research plan. Summaries from these meetings are included here for reference only.

WORKSHOP ON THE BIOLOGY OF CHROMOSOME 21 GENES: TOWARD THE GENE-PHENOTYPE CORRELATIONS IN DOWN SYNDROME, SEPTEMBER 2007

Dr. Katheleen Gardiner, the workshop organizer, welcomed the participants. She reminded the participants that three years had passed since the first expert workshop and that much has changed in the field of Down syndrome research internationally during that time.

Dr. Gardiner then provided an overview of the genes on human chromosome 21 (Hsa21). She presented a detailed description of the current state of knowledge of the 530 genes currently in the catalog for Hsa21, the level of their conservation among humans and mice, whether they encode microRNAs or functional RNAs, and their expected roles in various metabolic pathways. She summarized the current state of mouse models involving partial trisomies, their gene composition, and progress in creating models of triplication involving more of the genes triplicated in most humans with Down syndrome. Not only have investigators made progress identifying networks of interaction among genes, but investigators also recently identified polymorphisms that occur in genes located on Hsa21 that may have a substantial impact on comorbidities associated with Down syndrome, including dementia.

Dr. Dieressen then provided an overview of the Down syndrome phenotype, indicating that although John Langdon Down published his *Observations of the Ethnic Classification of Idiots* in 1866, Jean Étienne Esquirol authored the first attributable description of the condition in 1838. She alluded to the tremendous variability in both the phenotype that occurs and in the severity of the various aspects of the phenotypic spectrum. She described changes that occur in many organ systems as a result of Down syndrome and common effects on behavioral function. Dr. Dieressen also reviewed the structural changes in brain anatomy and physiology that may underlie these functional characteristics, emphasizing that changes in brain anatomy were not uniform, and that particular regions of the brain were particularly vulnerable developmentally in the trisomic state. Such changes may reflect alterations in the proliferation and survival of specific cell populations within those affected regions. Finally, she reminded the group that the postnatal environment during the first six months of life is very important, and that environmental enrichment during this critical period may have important and long-lasting effects on future cognitive function.

The first session, **Pathways and Processes I,** featured four presentations:

- The first focused on two *OLIG* genes, *OLIG1* and *OLIG2*, that control the development and maturation of not only oligodendrocytes, but also neurons.
- The next two presentations summarized studies of interactions involving the gene, *Intersectin*, with other genes, and its involvement not only in signal transduction and

endocytosis, but also its role in cell death and dendritic spine development, particularly spine elongation.

- The last presentation summarized studies of the interaction of the amyloid precursor protein fragment, Abeta, and its role in actin polymerization with *Rac1/CDC42 Rho GPTases* and *Tiam1*.

The second session, **Mouse Models I: Segmental Trisomies**, featured nine presentations. These presentations described newly developed mouse models relevant to the study of Down syndrome. Many of the presentations focused on comparative cellular and behavioral characteristics of these mice, their similarities to current models and importantly, their differences.

- The first discussed was the *Tc1* mouse, which contains an entire Hsa21, as an independent genetic unit (episome); these mice have some important differences in their phenotype.
- The second discussed the creation of mice trisomic for genes present on Hsa21, but located on other mouse chromosomes, Mmu17 and Mmu10; these mice have fewer of the features associated with previous mouse models.
- The third presentation discussed creation of a partially trisomic mouse, which contains the entire region of Mmu16 that is present on Hsa21; these mice have many peripheral features common to Down syndrome, including malformations of the cardiovascular and gastrointestinal systems. Unusual among partial trisomies in the mouse, these mice are viable and fertile on an inbred genetic background.
- The fourth discussed creation of partially trisomic mice using human artificial chromosomes engineered into mouse embryonic stem-cell lines; although the insertion is an episome, it is transmitted to each cell, unlike *Tc1*.
- The next three presentations focused on structural characteristics in partially trisomic mice, including those that have additional gene alterations, which permit examination of the role of specific genes on Mmu16 in cardiovascular and craniofacial development and in tumor repression. The results of these studies indicate that a number of effects on craniofacial and cardiovascular development associate with effects on neural crest-cell populations. Further, some males with *Ts65Dn* are fertile, making this model potentially more accessible to researchers as a whole. At least one gene, *Ets2*, plays an important role in solid tumor repression, and its dosage significantly affects tumor formation in both *Ts65Dn* and *Ts1Cje* mice.
- The next two presentations focused on hippocampal function.
  o The first discussed the role of *Girk2* in dysfunctional hippocampal inhibition.
  o The second discussed the role of the *App* gene in axonal transport of trophic factors on cholinergic neuron survival in the central nervous system, and on pain and temperature perception in the peripheral nervous system.

The third session, **Expression and Variation Symposium**, also featured nine presentations.

- Three presentations focused on comparative studies of RNA transcript levels and protein levels in a variety of tissues and cell lines derived from Down syndrome individuals.
  o One found that elevated protein levels did not accompany elevated RNA levels.
  o The second found variable, sometimes highly variable, levels of expression in blood cell lines with compensation occurring for more than half the genes studied.

- The third focused on studies of blood and skin cell lines; here dosage-sensitive overlapping genes may contribute to constant features of the phenotype, while partially overlapping genes contribute to more variable features.
- Three presentations focused discussion on studies of recombinant inbred mice and partially trisomic mice.
  - The first discussed direct comparison of each of the recombinant inbred mouse lines derived from one genetic inbred strain combination. Although a few genes were coordinately regulated, others correlated highly with specific cellular functions, like mitochondrial genes.
  - The second discussed similar studies of gene expression in *Ts65Dn* mice, in which broad variation occurred among individual mice and among brain regions. While specific gene expression was variable, some genes were under tight regulation in specific regions.
  - The third discussed structural changes to the cerebellum of the *Ts1Cj* mouse, in which only male mice are affected by changes in cerebellar volume and cell number. Further, a major gene dosage effect for only a few shared and differentially expressed genes may account for many of the cellular effects observed.
- Two presentations focused on studies of humans with partial trisomy 21.
  - The first described a new algorithm that allows resolution of breakpoints at the level of at least an exon and recording of actual copy number in high resolution comparative genomic hybridization (CGH) studies.
  - The second discussed a new customized Hsa21 CGH array that improves resolution significantly (at the gene level) over that of the current whole genome array.
- The last speaker, who was unable to attend, was to discuss genetic linkage between gastrointestinal phenotypes and leukemias in humans with partial trisomy 21.

The fourth session, **Chromosome 21 Gene Function**, featured nine presentations, including a number of "lightning" presentations derived from selected posters.
- Four presentations focused on studies of *RCAN1 (ADAPT78/DSCR1)* and other genes in the Down Syndrome Critical Region.
  - The first discussed the often antagonistic effects of different isoforms of *DSCR1* on cell stress, skeletal and cardiac muscle, and angiogenesis; these effects are mediated through effects on the calcineurin-NFAT pathways.
  - The second discussed the creation of transgenic mice, which overexpress human *RCAN1* under the control of a neuron-specific *enolase* promoter and described the resulting altered behavior. Disruption of vascular development and tone in mice transgenic for *RCAN1* in all tissues led to prenatal lethality due to hemorrhage, while knockout mice exhibited altered nitric oxide production.
  - The third discussed the essential role of the Down Syndrome Cell Adhesion Molecule, DSCAM, a homophilic cell-adhesion molecule, in commissural axon guidance.
  - The fourth discussed the role of *Dyrk1A* overexpression in cognitive abnormalities; here premature exit of progenitors from the expansive phase of the cell cycle results in generation of fewer neurons.

- Another presentation discussed ectopic expression of the *Autoimmune Regulator-Expressing (AIRE)* gene in transformed thymic epithelia cells in culture and its role in cell adhesion and apoptosis.
- One presentation discussed the role of the mammalian *Mre11* complex in the genesis of aneuploidy. Aneuploidy is normally a rare event in mice, but mutations in *Mre11* significantly alter homologous recombination in a sex-dependent manner by causing premature separation of chromosomes and random segregation
- Two presentations discussed microRNAs encoded on Hsa21:
  - The first identified the microRNAs shared on Hsa21 and Mmu16 and discussed how the study of available partially trisomic mouse models could facilitate elucidation of the role of specific mRNAs in the control of translation.
  - The second focused on one specific microRNA, *has-miR-155*, and its role in vascular blood pressure through interaction with the gene *AGTR*; here polymorphisms of a specific nucleotide are associated with hypertension, and overexpression lowers blood pressure.
- The final presentation compared ENCODE, which focuses on all functional elements in 1 percent of the human genome with GENCODE, which focuses on all coding genes. ENCODE enables isolation of novel exons that show some conservation in the mammalian lineage. Further, 40 percent of tandem genes produce chimeric transcripts that may be functional, an unexpected finding.

The fifth session, **Analysis of Protein Expression**, featured three presentations:
- The first outlined the increasing use of bioinformatics analysis of genomic and proteomic databases to determine the roles of gene in nervous system function, and how selective depletion of common components of sera can generate completely different constellations of proteins for study.
- The second focused on using MALDI MS to detect expression of *PEP-19* in tissue section of mouse brain; the effects of treatment of striatum with specific neurotoxic drugs; and comparison resulting profiles with the *SwePep* database for bioactive, partially bioactive, and uncharacterized peptides.
- The third focused on models of traumatic brain injury and methods available to assay subsets of differentially expressed proteins, proteins undergoing proteolytic truncation or fragmentation, and interactive protein pathways.

The sixth session, **Pathways and Processes II**, also featured three presentations related to the calcineurin pathway.
- The first discussed the interaction of *DSCR1/RCAN1/MCIP1* expression with circadian clock-gene expression in several peripheral tissues and the suprachiasmatic nucleus, and its additional effect on innate circadian day length, and the use of CreSCN-specific transgenic mice to further elucidate the role of calcineurin in this process.
- The second discussed how expression of *Dyrk1a* affects phosphorylation to regulate endocytic protein interactions, and how synaptic activity may alter binding with the participation of calcium/calcineurin and ionotropic glutamate receptors.
- The third described characteristics of lines of transgenic mice harboring mutations in NFATc transcription factors and their similarities to partially trisomic mice and mice that overexpress *Dyrk1a* and *Dscr1*.

The seventh session, **Mouse Models II – Single Genes**, featured eight presentations:

- Three presentations related to single genes in the calcineurin pathway. The first related increased phosphorylation of APP and Tau in BAC transgenic mice expressing h*DYRK1A* in elevated levels of beta-amyloid and learning deficits. The second compared *RCAN1* and *Rcan1* null transgenic mice with respect to retrograde transport, hippocampal volume, cell size, and dendritic spine number, and behavioral performance. The third related mice lacking *Mcip1* expression to mice overexpressing calcineurin with respect to behavior and electrophysiological characteristics. Generation of conditional transgenics selectively targeting pyramidal neurons in forebrain and specific hippocampal regions should allow further study of alternations in the calcineurin pathway.
- Two presentations discussed the role of specific genes in endocytotic pathway function. The first related the role of *Intersectin (ITSN1)* in cholinergic neuron survival and trophic transport in *ITSN1* null mice, alterations that also affect endocytotic pathways in their chromaffin cells. The second studied both *Ts65Dn* mice and mice overexpressing *synaptojanin 1* (*Synj1*), a lipid phosphatase and found increased phosphatase activity correlated with behavioral learning deficits.
- Three presentations related derivatives of ectoderm and neural crest cells in peripheral tissues, and neurons. The first discussed overexpression of *PCP4* (*PEP19*) in mice with either the mouse or human gene. Overexpression led to precocious cell differentiation in a cell line and altered dendritic branching in the brain. The second discussed changes that take place in the skin of mice transgenic for *hSOD1* and *hAPP*, as well as *Ts1Cje* mice; changes that may result from significant changes in detoxification enzymes as a result of oxidative stress. The third discussed the use of mutagenesis screens to detect novel loci that affect neural crest development in mice.

The eighth session, **Pathways and Processes III**, featured three presentations that related oxidative stress and mitochondrial dysfunction:

- The first discussed the myriad of structural and functional effects that changes in mitochondrial structure and function have in the nervous system. Study of Neurospheres, blood cell precursors, and fetal pancreatic cells all revealed reduced proliferation. Although treatment with creatine rescued the phenotype, it did not restore function.
- The second discussed the frequent occurrence of a specific mutation, *T414G*, in the somatic mitochondrial DNA control region in blood cells from individuals with dementia due to Alzheimer disease or Down syndrome.
- The third discussed several Has 21 genes that are critical to the pathogenesis of both *Herpes* and *Coxsackie B* viruses and the lethal vascular consequences to mice lacking the receptor for the *Coxsackie B* receptor.

The ninth session, **The Potential for Therapeutics**, featured six presentations focused on pharmacologic, dietary, and gene therapy interventions in mice, dogs, and humans.

- The first discussed the use of oral feeding of phenylenetetrazone to improve learning and memory in *Ts65Dn* mice, an improvement that persisted for several months after drug discontinuation.
- The second focused on the use of memantine to mimic the effects of calcineurin on the learning behavior of *Ts65Dn* mice.

- The third used prenatal and postnatal dietary intervention with epigallocatechin gallate, an ingredient of green tea, to reverse the effects of overexpression of *Dyrk1a* in YAC transgenic mice. This intervention also improved expression of the neurotrophin, BDNF.
- A fourth discussed targeting the interferon system with Normoferon during embryogenesis, with dramatic improvement in transgenic and trisomic mice.
- The fifth discussed the direct use of adenoassociated viral gene therapy using shRNA injections into the striatum to improve behavior and motor performance of *Dyrk1a* transgenic mice.
- The final presentation presented the results of two antioxidant dietary studies, one in dogs and one in humans, on progression of dementia. The discussion underscored the need for consistent measures across study groups and the usefulness of telecommunications in recruiting more subjects to clinical studies.

Group Discussion

Dr. Gardiner began the discussion by highlighting several immediate needs: moving from animal to human studies; developing a clinical network; and moving animal experimentation to therapies. The research community needs standardized evaluation to screen compounds. The community needs to relate tests in animals to tests in humans, after repeating experiments done in one model in several laboratories and then in several different models. The community needs to promote available models and to share what investigators did to get their results, so that others can replicate them. The current status of animal availability and limited sources for distribution hampers efforts of the research community. Recently, directors of various Down syndrome clinics in the United States formed a Down Syndrome Interest Group that meets annually to develop a strategy to create a centralized database and facilitate data sharing, possibly by combining samples into a central repository for access by interested investigators.

Others in the audience emphasized the need for resources and clinical trials networks. Some felt that researchers needed to go into the community to "set the record straight" about the current status of Down syndrome research and, importantly, about the need for the alternative medicine clinical trials, which some proposed for use by individuals with Down syndrome based on anecdotal evidence. Others emphasized the importance of medical compliance because even available medications are useless if they are not taken. Further, in individuals who live independent from family or in a structured living environment, as many as one in three may miss their medications routinely.

The research community needs to agree on a set of common tests to apply to the various mouse models in a consistent manner. A panel of tests that would differentiate hippocampal function from prefrontal cortex function would be very useful. There is also need for a panel of neurocognitive tests investigators can use across laboratories. When investigators collect clinical samples, a central storage facility would make the samples easily available to future researchers.

In Europe, a consortium of researchers have come to consensus concerning behavioral tests to apply, brain regions to collect, and storage of samples and data in a common repository. Because a carefully defined natural history of cognitive development in Down syndrome is lacking, it is difficult to develop testing tools that probe the cognitive strengths and weaknesses of Down syndrome individuals adequately. The research community needs to create that body of data and might consider evaluation of the standard tests developed by Nadel to determine the abilities and the variability among individuals with Down syndrome and within these individuals over time. The research community needs to develop robust measures.

Parents in the audience pointed out that the school systems, through the Individuals with Disabilities Education Act (IDEA), annually gave cognitive tests to students. Better communication between the lay public and the research communities would facilitate exchange of information between the groups and the formation of a workforce partnership. The parents present emphasized the need for improved performance for their children, not for more funding of prenatal and newborn screening. They needed therapeutic interventions, not diagnostics.

Dr. Oster-Granite from the NICHD made a presentation on the current status of the NIH Down Syndrome Working Group and its efforts and provided information concerning the sources of recommendations from various meetings, panels of experts, and various advocacy groups. She added that the draft of a research plan mandated by Congress would be available for public comment in the imminent future. She requested that members of the audience read the report and provide their comments as soon as possible.

The issue of the number and availability of antibodies for research studies prompted Dr. Riddle from the NINDS to explain that NINDS and NIMH currently fund a project at the University of California, Davis, to produce monoclonal antibodies for nervous system specific genes. Investigators in the Down syndrome research community could make use of this service to generate antibodies for each of the genes on Hsa21. A current NIH Blueprint for Neuroscience Research solicitation may be of interest as well.

Because Down syndrome is an international condition, one individual suggested that perhaps an international consortium could adopt international models, and that the United States might benefit from the model created by the European Union. Others pointed out that comparisons are often difficult because the various mouse models exist on different genetic backgrounds to enable reproduction.

Posters

The following posters received formal platform presentations at the meeting:
- *Human MicroRNA-155 on Chromosome 21 Differentially Interacts with Its Polymorphic Target in the AFTR1 3' Untranslated Region: A Mechanism for Functional Single-Nucleotide Polymorphisms Related to Phenotypes*
- *Trisomy 21 Murine Models and Skin Pathologies*
- *The Mammalian Mre11 Complex Plays an Important Role in Homologous Recombination*
- *The Involvement of RCAN1 (ADAPT78/DSCR1) in Down Syndrome*
- *PCP4 (PEP19) Overexpression: Consequences of One Additional Gene Copy on Neuronal Differentiation in* in vitro *and* in vivo *Models of Down Syndrome*
- *SYNJ1-Linked PtdIns(4,5)P2 Dyshomeostasis and Cognitive Deficits in Mouse Models of Down Syndrome*
- *Elucidating the Role of RCAN1/DSCR1 in Brain Development and Function*

- *Altered Mitochondrial Function and Secretory Defects in Down Syndrome Pancreatic Precursor Cells*
- *Production of Novel Down Syndrome Mouse Model Using Human Artificial Chromosome (HAC)*
- *Vesicle Trafficking and BFCN: Abnormalities in ITSN1 Null Mice*
- *Characterization of an Aneuploid Mouse with a Human Chromosome that Models Down Syndrome*
- *Overexpression of Dyrk1A Affects Proliferation and Differentiation of Neural Progenitor Cells*

The following posters provided additional information not discussed by the participants in oral presentations.

- *AnEUploidy: Understanding Gene Dosage Imbalance in Human Health.* The overall goal of this integrated project involving 17 laboratories in 19 European countries is to understand the molecular mechanisms of gene dosage imbalance in human health, using genetics, functional genomics, and systems biology.
- The authors of *Mapping of Small RNAs in the Human Encode Regions (Including Chromosome 21)* described the mapping of size fractionated RNAs, particularly small RNA fragments, by forward and reverse ENCODE high-density resolution tiling arrays.
- The authors of *Sprouty2 Inhibitory Activity on FGF-Signaling is Modulated by the Protein Kinase DYRK1A* described the interaction of *DYRK1A* and *Sprouty2*, whose coexpression in appropriate neuronal populations affects the FGF-MAPK pathway close to early activation events to ensure appropriate neuronal cell response to growth factors.
- The authors of *Dyrk1A is Involved in Neuronal Survival during Development of the Central Nervous System* found that *Dyrk1A +/-* mice exhibit a significant reduction in brain size and in the numbers of retinal ganglion and mesencephalic dopaminergic neurons, but not serotoninergic neurons. Increased apoptosis accounts for the cell number change, since the numbers of neurons generated is the same at midgestation.
- The authors of *Spatial Learning Impairment in Mice Haploinsufficient for the Dual Specificity Tyrosine-Regulated Kinase-1A (Dyrk1A)* describe the use of the Morris water maze to test both hippocampal-dependent and hippocampal-independent learning and memory, as well as a swim test, and a test of floating behavior in water at two different temperatures to study cognitive function and stress coping behavior in *Dyrk1A+/-* mice. They found significant impairment in spatial learning-hippocampal dependent memory task, increased sensitivity to aversive conditions, and increased hypothermia-induced floating behavior.
- The authors of *Down Syndrome Mouse Models and the Response to the NMDA Antagonist MK801* describe studies in both *Ts65Dn* and *Ts1Cje* mice treated with MK801. They found treatment dependent abnormalities in activation and/or localization of critical pathway components, including pAkt, pErk1/2, and pGSK3B, plus the transcription factor Elk, and proteins TIAM1 and DYRK1A. Treatment affects basal levels of protein activity and dynamics of responses to stimuli. .
- The authors of *The Potential Involvement of RCAN1 (ADAPT78/DSCR1)-Mediated Vasoregulation in Down Syndrome* describe the basis for the mesenteric artery vasoconstriction observed in *Rcan1* knockout mice, elevated nitric oxide through

inhibition of calcineurin. The use of L-NAME, a NOS inhibitor, produces a similar effect, altering blood flow and blood vessel development.

- The authors of *Analysis of CBS Expression in Transgenic Mice for the Human CBS (Cystathionine Beta Synthase) Gene* describe studies of mice who express only the human *CBS* gene. They found decreased levels of homocysteine, but increased levels of hydrogen sulfide. They examined CBS expression in several brain regions and in the liver. Concomitant with increased expression, they found a 30-percent increase in enzyme levels. In these mice, the human gene under its own promoter does not follow same expression as mouse gene.

- The authors of *Alzheimer Disease-Like Pathology in a Murine Model Overexpressing Dyrk1A, a Gene Involved in Down Syndrome* describe their studies of aged (22 month to 25 month) versus adult (6 month to 8 month) *Dyrk1A* overexpressing mice. They found an age associated impairment in recent memory that involved the cholinergic system.

- The authors of *A Humanized Mouse Model for the Reduced Folate Carrier* produced *TghRFC1* mice and humanized mice with *mRFC* inactivated. They found that specificity of expression closely resembles that observed in human tissues.

- The authors of *RCAN1 Increases Neuronal Susceptibility to Oxidative Stress: A Potential Pathogenic Process in Neurodegeneration* found RCAN was sensitive to oxidative stress in cerebellar granule cells. In *Rcan1 -/-* mice, the authors observed an increased resistance to hydrogen peroxide that they could reverse by using inhibitors of calcineurin.

- The authors of a *Role of Oxidative Stress in CREB Dysregulation in Ts65Dn Mouse Brain* describe a significant decrease in CREB-mediated transcription of BDNF in *Ts65Dn* mouse brain. They found that overexpression *CREB* decreased neuronal apoptosis. They observed that, at eight months, *Ts65Dn* mice exhibited significantly decreased phosphorylated CREB in the hippocampus, but increased levels in cerebellum. This finding coincided with increased levels of GFAP in the hippocampus, but not in the cerebellum.

- The authors of *The Effects of Ets2 on the Craniofacial Skeleton in Down Syndrome* describe differences in skull development in *Ts65DnEts2+/-* mice. Although they found that effects in both mesoderm-derived and neural crest-derived skeletal elements in *Ts65Dn* mice and in *Ts65DnEts2+/-* mice, the effects in *Ts65DnEts2+/-* mice were significantly different for neural crest-derived skeletal elements.

- The authors of *Cellular and Molecular "Common Denominators" to Down Syndrome Phenotype*s describe the use of cultures of pharyngeal arch 1 to examine the role of *Sonic hedgehog (Shh)* expression on cell proliferation. They found, as they had previously observed in the cerebellum and skull of *Ts65Dn* mice, reduced cellular proliferation of the mandibular anlagen. Treatment of the cultures with *Shh* overcame deficits in cell proliferation, providing direct evidence that Down syndrome is a neurocrestopathy.

MEETING ON FACTORS THAT AFFECT COGNITIVE FUNCTION IN DOWN SYNDROME THROUGHOUT THE LIFESPAN, JULY 2007

Sponsored by the NICHD on behalf of the NIH Down Syndrome Working Group, the meeting gathered researchers and other experts from around the country (including representatives from key federal agencies and national organizations that focus on Down syndrome) to discuss *Factors that Affect Cognitive Function in Down Syndrome Throughout the Lifespan.* As stated during opening comments, the purpose of the meeting was to gather input and recommendations from the scientific field on various aspects of research relating to Down syndrome, in preparation for development of the research plan by NIH.

Two opening presentations set the stage for more specific discussions of recommendations for research goals. Dr. Marilyn Field provided an overview of a new report (April 2007) from the Institute of Medicine, *The Future of Disability in America,* which took a broad look at what progress has been made in understanding disability, its causes, and ways to prevent its onset or progression. The report included a particular focus on aging with a disability and transitions from pediatric to adult health care, both issues of concern for individuals with Down syndrome and their families. Dr. Charles Epstein provided an historical perspective on research during the past 160 years relevant to Down syndrome; he also described the basic phenotype of people with Down syndrome, and its variability. He touched upon aging and genetic issues as emerging topics for research.

Each speaker at the meeting was asked to include their recommendations for future research needs in their particular areas of expertise. The first group of experts discussed research directions and needs for the areas of genomics and proteomics. Although a large number of proteomic approaches are available to help identify what proteins may be changing, several presenters highlighted the need for scientists to better understand how mice differ from humans; they noted that these differences must be elucidated to determine which research questions can be answered using Down syndrome mouse models, and which require human subjects. Similarly, a fundamental issue in using mouse models was the need to determine which genetic situations in mice were analogous to those in humans. Even though the *Tc1* mouse model contains a nearly intact copy of human chromosome 21, some gaps still exist. Current research aims to identify gene clusters in individuals with Down syndrome that may account for the variations. Other research is progressing with a focus on the neurotrophic factor (NTF) hypothesis and its application to Down syndrome research; the hypothesis states that target-driven NTFs are required for the survival and differentiation of neurons. Further research is needed on NTF signals to see if any signaling defect in Down syndrome can be detected. During the discussion that followed, the group generally seemed to agree that while a great deal of research effort has focused on developing and refining models relevant to Down syndrome, the availability and cost of obtaining these models has prevented the field from advancing as quickly as might be possible. In addition, discussants noted that the field needs a coherent mouse model analysis program that would permit the development of a battery of standardized behaviors.

The presentations on the subject of medical issues that affect cognitive function in children and adolescents with Down syndrome focused on changes in development and cognitive function as children grow into adulthood, and on comorbidities; at least half of all children with Down syndrome have a comorbid condition. A number of these conditions, including congenital heart disease, hypoxic-ischemic encephalopathy, seizure disorders, psychiatric or neurobehavioral problems, sleep apnea and other sleep disturbances, hearing loss, and childhood leukemias, may affect cognition and, in turn, affect treatment. Outcomes are also not uniform; some research shows that when children with a genetic disorder have heart surgery, they have much poorer neurodevelopmental outcomes than children without such disorders.

A range of behavioral and psychosocial factors affect cognitive function throughout the lifespan of a person with Down syndrome. Early behavioral interventions are being tested to improve quality of life for these individuals and their families, not to cure the intellectual disability of Down syndrome itself, but to increase skills and functional levels. The benefits of certain compensatory strategies, such as language interventions that assist in processing linguistic input, must be tested more thoroughly, and more should be identified. Concerning families' reactions to family members who have Down syndrome, researchers have begun to recognize that not all the effects of having a child with disabilities are negative; parents and siblings of children with Down syndrome often report experiencing less stress than families of children with other disabilities. At the same time, more work is needed, including efforts in the areas of the demographics of families of children with Down syndrome, family reactions to a child's personal characteristics, and measuring other real-world outcomes for the family, such as stress. Because children with Down syndrome live longer lives, presenters recommended more research on the intergenerational transmission of caregiving responsibilities. Along those lines, another presenter noted that the aging process might have an accelerated impact on cognition in Down syndrome and suggested longitudinal studies to address this and related issues.

Another portion of the program highlighted recent or ongoing animal and human clinical trials related to Down syndrome. A national trial of antioxidants in beagle dogs explored the oxidative stress hypothesis, showing a sustained improvement in cognitive function and several biomarkers for oxidative stress, particularly when combined with environmental enrichment. A series of clinical studies of NMDA-receptor antagonist in people with moderate to severe Alzheimer disease showed that the drug produced a small increase in neurocognitive ability that warranted further study. Vitamin E has also shown some promise in slowing deterioration. Another line of work showed that women with Down syndrome, who experience menopause earlier than other women, may receive a protective effect against dementia if they take hormone replacement therapy. Statins are also being discussed to help people with Down syndrome, who usually have higher cholesterol levels, decrease their risk of dementia. Presenters mentioned a number of promising technologies that are on the horizon, including the use of the new Positron Emission Tomography (PET) ligands and magnetic resonance spectroscopy to study neuron health, and a range of treatments already being tested in the Alzheimer disease community.

Meeting participants broke into subgroups to consolidate and list their suggestions for how to move the Down syndrome research and technology field forward. The Research Infrastructure group recommended the establishment of a standing committee composed of NIH representatives, extramural scientists, and community members to manage and guide the NIH Down syndrome research portfolio, including oversight of a new mouse virtual core (to increase availability of mouse models), validation of models for Down syndrome research, clinical trials, and proteomics. The group added that the national Down syndrome organizations could be particularly helpful in encouraging participation in research, especially recruitment for clinical trials, and in encouraging donation of tissues. The needs for a national registry/database, and a champion within NIH to speak for Down syndrome research were also identified.

The Behavioral and Family Issues group noted that the most significant impacts on the behavioral and cognitive profiles of people with Down syndrome have come from planned interventions and policy changes. New research on interventions using the family, school, and home environments was recommended, as was research on ways to enhance physical fitness. A strong plea was made to focus research on people with Down syndrome and their families, as opposed to only using this group as controls for research on other conditions. In addition, researchers noted the need for cognitive, language, and behavior measures for use across the lifespan because those appropriate for one stage of life are not appropriate for others.

The Medical Issues group led with the suggestion that the NIH develop pediatric Down syndrome collaborative centers or networks to study the condition and its associated aspects. These centers could conduct research, including longitudinal studies and clinical trials, offer training, and develop new research tools. This last suggestion was echoed by the Clinical Trials group, which noted the need for well-trained clinical trials specialists with experience in the condition, and the need for mechanisms to screen new therapeutic agents for efficacy.

GATLINBURG CONFERENCE, MARCH 2007

(Note: This workshop report summarizes the presentations and discussions of research gaps made during the workshop.)

The Gatlinburg Conference represents one of the premier conferences in the United States for behavioral scientists conducting research in intellectual and related developmental disabilities. The theme for the 2007 Conference was *Down Syndrome: Genes, Brain, and Behavior.*

Down syndrome is the leading genetic cause of intellectual disability. Moreover, research on Down syndrome displays a level of "maturity" as regards the multidisciplinary approaches investigators have developed to study the causal pathways from genes to behavior. These approaches include animal models that investigators have phenotyped in considerable detail, stem cells used to study the earliest stages of neural development at a cellular level, innovative neuroimaging studies that have documented anatomical differences, psychometrically sophisticated approaches to the measurement of behavior, behavioral change related to age and in response to environmental variations, and epidemiological studies that have tracked changes in prevalence and the societal conditions responsible for those changes. Investigators can use Down syndrome as a model for planning investigations into less well-understood genetic conditions associated with intellectual disability.

This year's theme for the Gatlinburg conference reflected this multidisciplinary approach to understanding Down syndrome, with invited speakers representing approaches that are perhaps less familiar to the regular attendees of the conference, thereby enriching and expanding both conceptual and methodological repertoires. Presentations on this theme came from all disciplines relevant to understanding the causes, consequences, life-course trajectories, and environmental circumstances.

Four plenary sessions provided the participants with the opportunity to hear internationally recognized Down syndrome researchers from the biomedical and behavioral fields. Dr. Stephanie Sherman presented *Trisomy 21: Causes and Consequences*. Dr. Sherman discussed the results of her long-standing study of the epidemiological factors associated with Down syndrome and summarized her recent study conducted in collaboration with the Centers for Disease Control and Prevention (CDC) and the Down Syndrome Registry, a six-state epidemiological study. These factors include the source of the nondisjunction event as the mother (93 percent) and the well-established effect of maternal age (35 percent older than age 40). The incidence of Down syndrome remains quite stable (1:732) across populations sampled in six states, although Hispanics have a higher prevalence ratio (1.11) and African Americans a lower ratio (0.78) than Caucasians. The type of error that occurs is associated with exchanges at specific regions along the chromosome during meiosis. This is more likely to be telomeric for meiosis 1 errors (which happen during the intrauterine life of the mother) and pericentromeric for meiosis II errors. Meiosis II errors are also maternal-age dependent. Congenital heart disease is a common feature and may occur in up to 50 percent of liveborn infants with Down syndrome. There is, however, racial disparity in the incidence of particular defects, the most frequent of which is atrioventricular septal defect. Its frequency among African Americans is 35 percent, but among Hispanics only 12 percent. Specific DNA markers associate with the African American population that exhibit congenital heart disease. A limited oocyte pool also associates with both advanced maternal age or with ovariectomy and increases the risk of meiotic errors and slightly decreases the age of menopause. Maternal age increases the risk of recurrence among those older than age 30.

Dr. Ira Lott presented *Down Syndrome and Alzheimer Disease: Clues from Neuroimaging*. Dr. Lott discussed his considerable experience with the onset of dementia and its clinical course in individuals with Down syndrome. Although the course of progression of Alzheimer disease in the general population is between 10 and 15 years, it may be as rapid as 3 to 4 years in individuals with Down syndrome. The neuropathologic characteristics of Alzheimer disease are ubiquitous by age 40 and may appear in the first decade of life. Even though there is evidence of premature aging in Down syndrome, there is virtually no incidence of atherosclerotic stroke or hypertension. Pre-demented Down syndrome individuals exhibit an increased glucose metabolic signal in entorhinal cortex and a decreased signal in the cingulate gyrus, while individuals who develop Alzheimer disease exhibit a decreased signal in both areas. Changes in glucose metabolism in Down syndrome individuals may be predictive of the onset of dementia. Dr. Lott also discussed the results of trials of combined antioxidants (vitamins E and C, carnitine, and alpha lipoic acid) in beagles. In the presence of an enriched environment, the beagles neither improved nor worsened. In a human clinical trial of Down syndrome individuals with dementia, administration of vitamins E and C with alpha lipoic acid led to very little change in the treated group, but the placebo group experienced a rapid acceleration in decline. Elevated cholesterol levels also associate with an increased incidence of dementia; treatment with statins reduced the risk by 60 percent in individuals with Down syndrome. In females with Down syndrome, early menopause associates with earlier development of dementia. Dr. Lott described how he uses telemedicine to rapidly diagnose patients with the onset of dementia.

Dr. Jennifer Wishart presented *Social Cognition in Children with Down Syndrome: Current Evidence, Future Directions.* She discussed the results of her studies during the past two decades, indicating that early intervention did not provide clear results of usefulness because often the interventions were not targeted to strengths or weaknesses. Few individuals with Down syndrome develop adequate communication skills, and language development is delayed over and above what one might expect for a given IQ. Down syndrome affects all domains of communication and one needs to use a developmental approach to the problems. Progress often takes longer and is not synchronous, so there is the expectation of low learning in children with Down syndrome. Often Down syndrome children use avoidance strategies and misuse social skills. Although emotional recognition appears early, children with Down syndrome can do these visual recognition tests, but not as well as other children. Children with Down syndrome may benefit from using peer partners to learn and in cooperative learning situations, rather than in collaborative learning situations.

Dr. Roger Reeves presented *Therapy for Structural Abnormalities in the Trisomic Brain*, and discussed the substantial progress made in treatment strategies in animal model systems. These strategies may apply to individuals with Down syndrome. The first is the observation that treatment of the most commonly studied mouse model of Down syndrome with the GABAa antagonist, pentylenetetrazole, normalized their responses, and this effect persisted for months after treatment. However, this medication is associated with increased incidence of seizures in humans, making it problematic as a medication for Down syndrome. Other GABAa antagonists may however have few adverse effects in humans and would benefit from trial in mouse models. Alteration of the overexpression of the gene encoding the amyloid precursor protein (APP) through mating partially trisomic *Ts65Dn* mice with *APP-/+* mice restored NGF transport in basal forebrain cholinergic neurons and enabled their continued survival. Thus, three copies of *APP* in individuals with Down syndrome affect the survival of cholinergic neurons. The use of the mitogenic Sonic hedgehog agonist, SAG, increased proliferation of cerebellar granule cells in *Ts65Dn* mice and enabled more normal cerebellar development and foliation.

Several symposia focused specifically on Down syndrome. The first, *Down Syndrome, Aging, and Alzheimer Disease: Practical Insights from Prospective Studies*, presented data from a longitudinal cohort study spanning two decades. Presenters discussed such topics as the relationship of elevated amyloid-beta-peptide and its association with the incidence of dementia and mortality, the association of the apolipoprotein E epsilon 4 isoform with increased mortality in Down syndrome individuals who are not demented, mild cognitive impairment in adults, and the effectiveness of treatment with cholinesterase inhibitors in adults. Another session, *Selective Neuropsychological Changes Across the Adult Lifespan in Down Syndrome*, featured presentations on declines in visual-spatial abilities in young adults, visual-spatial working memory decline associated with mild cognitive impairment and dementia, and neuropathological evidence of Alzheimer disease in Down syndrome.

The session, *Siblings of Individuals with Developmental Disabilities Across the Lifespan*, included a presentation on parent-sibling communication in families of children with autism, Down syndrome, and sickle-cell disease. Another, *Children with Down Syndrome: Parent and Child Supports*, included presentations on parent-child communication at homes with preschool children having Down syndrome and autism, coping with frustration in children, and examining parental stress and parental perceptions of toddler communication development following language intervention. On a similar theme, the session *Phenotypic Responses to Communication Intervention in Young Children with Down Syndrome* focused on treatment (non)effects and predictors of communication and language development, responses of children to prelinguistic milieu teaching, and the effects of early augmented language intervention on communication skills.

The session, *Down Syndrome: Gene Expression and Beyond*, covered the function of chromosome 21 gene products in *bacterial artificial chromosome* (*BAC*)-transgenic mice, the role of the PIP2 phosphatase synaptojanin 1 in brain dysfunction, and the consequences of overexpression of the gene minibrain (*Mnb/Dyrk1A*).

Approaching the issue from another public health front, the session *What Large-Scale Administrative Databases Can Tell Us about Down Syndrome*, featured presentations on the use of administrative databases, the demography of births with Down syndrome in Tennessee, adverse birth outcomes in Down syndrome, and the use of propensity scores to match multiple variables in Down syndrome.

In addition, two poster sessions and one paper session focused on Down syndrome. The first featured the work of investigators who study persistence in early communication by young children with Down syndrome, factors that predict mortality for individuals who reside in a family, enhancing cognitive-emotional skills through computer-based training, special health care needs, teaching money skills, developmental trajectories in language skills, parental coping assistance, maternal responsiveness characteristics in Fragile X and Down syndromes, and life events and psychological outcomes. Investigators are also studying depression and well-being in mothers, mediators of stress in parents, family cohesion and its influence on adaptive behavior, auditory responses in newborns with Down syndrome, maternal experience of bereavement in parents of children with Down syndrome and congenital heart disease, and understanding the causes of emotions by others in children with Down syndrome.

A paper session, *Down Syndrome and Interventions*, featured presentations on telomere shortening in individuals with Down syndrome and dementia; Down syndrome, aging, and Alzheimer disease; using electropalatography to assess speech articulation difficulties in children with Down syndrome; inclusive education and social isolation among adolescents with Down syndrome; and establishing building blocks of cognitive behavior therapy.

OUTREACH MEETING WITH RESEARCH ADVOCACY ORGANIZATIONS, DECEMBER 2006

The NICHD and the NIH Down Syndrome Working Group hosted a meeting with representatives of key research advocacy organizations, whose missions relate to Down syndrome, that form the Down Syndrome Research Coalition to share their respective plans for encouraging research in this area. The Coalition is preparing its own National Research Agenda, but wanted to meet with the federal agencies involved to coordinate their recommendations. Ultimately, the Coalition's goal is to establish federal partnerships for each of their major research goals.

The meeting also provided an opportunity for the Coalition to hear from many of the NIH Institutes and Centers about the research they support on many aspects of Down syndrome, and the scientific meetings planned over the next year, including the Gatlinburg Conference, an NIH-sponsored conference to gather input on the research plan, and a meeting funded by the NICHD focusing on the genes present on chromosome 21.

Looking forward, the entire group also discussed how to disseminate the various research plans and other relevant information throughout the scientific, patient/family, and research advocacy communities. The NIH Office of Research Services will conduct a literature search and make it available to meeting participants. In addition, the group considered the possibility of an entire journal issue devoted to Down syndrome research.

WORKSHOP ON DOWN SYNDROME: TOWARD OPTIMAL SYNAPTIC FUNCTION AND COGNITION, FEBRUARY 2005

(Note: The following is the official published workshop report, which summarizes the presentations and discussions of research gaps made during the workshop. See http://www.ninds.nih.gov/news_and_events/proceedings/down_sydrome_2005.htm.)

Down syndrome is the most common genetic cause of mental retardation, occurring in 1 in 800 live births. Down syndrome patients suffer not only cognitive deficits, but also early onset Alzheimer disease, facial dysmorphology, and increased frequencies of congenital heart disease, gastrointestinal anomalies, and leukemia. Nevertheless, the life expectancy of Down syndrome individuals has improved greatly during the past 30 years, to an average of more than 50 years. As the life expectancy of Down syndrome individuals increases, their intellectual disabilities and early onset dementia pose increasing personal and societal burdens.

Despite the prevalence of Down syndrome, relatively little research has been devoted to understanding the biology of this syndrome, or to developing therapeutics. This neglect has been due, in part, to the presumed global nature of the molecular and cellular abnormalities in Down syndrome: the syndrome is caused by trisomy for chromosome 21, and hence involves misexpression of hundreds of genes. Recent work in mouse models of Down syndrome suggests that there are a variety mechanisms of gene action behind the multitude of phenotypic effects of trisomy 21; for some phenotypes, a very few individual genes on chromosome 21 may be particularly critical. In addition, specific synaptic defects have now been identified in mouse models of Down syndrome that appear to be amenable to pharmacological correction. The goal of this workshop was to review recent advances in Down syndrome research and relevant technical approaches to identify key priority areas for future work. The invited participants included not only leaders in the field of Down syndrome research, but also basic neuroscientists not currently working on Down syndrome whose future involvement might help propel the field.

Overview of Cognitive Deficits in Down Syndrome

There is a specific pattern of cognitive deficits in Down syndrome that differs from that seen in other mental retardation syndromes (such as Fragile X or Williams syndrome). People with Down syndrome have relatively high levels of social intelligence, but are impaired in expressive communication and explicit memory. Sleep problems are also frequent and may exacerbate the memory problems. Interestingly, the cognitive functions most affected are subserved by structures that mature relatively late in development, such as the prefrontal cortex, hippocampus, and cerebellum.

In addition to the defects in cognitive development that become evident early in life, another major feature of Down syndrome is an early onset dementia of the Alzheimer's type. Many patients start showing symptoms of Alzheimer's by early middle age, and few are spared completely. It is unclear to what extent the processes underlying the development of the dementia overlap with those responsible for the defects seen in cognitive development. There is also a mysterious variability in the age of onset of dementia in Down syndrome: some patients start showing signs in their early 40s, while others appear unaffected even in their 60s and 70s. The genetic factors responsible for the variable penetrance of the dementia phenotype have not yet been explored, but could prove highly informative about the biology of both Down syndrome and Alzheimer disease.

RECOMMENDATIONS:
1. Catalog more precisely the cognitive deficits that occur in Down syndrome, through neuropsychological testing and functional imaging, and in both children and adults. This effort would enable identification of circuits that might be targeted for eventual therapeutics, as well as identify key deficits for study in animal models.

2. Create a DNA repository for patients with Down syndrome to enable genotype/phenotype analyses on: (1) the nature and severity of cognitive deficits; and (2) the age of onset and severity of dementia.

Synapse Formation and Structure

A number of developmental abnormalities have been described in the brains of individuals with Down syndrome. By 18 months postnatal, abnormalities in the development of dendritic spines are seen: spine density is decreased, and spines that are either larger or thinner than normal have been reported. Dendritic abnormalities are also seen in mice that model Down syndrome, where increases in spine size are seen throughout the brain and a decrease in spine density is seen in the hippocampus. Such abnormalities are consistent with the memory deficits seen in human Down syndrome, and with abnormalities in synaptic plasticity (i.e., long-term potentiation) seen in

Down syndrome model mice. A number of synaptic proteins may be up- or down-regulated in Down syndrome that are critical to normal spine development and synapse formation.

A key unanswered question is whether defects in synaptic development are initiators of the development of the Down syndrome cognitive phenotype, or whether they are a secondary consequence of other, possibly earlier problems in development. For example, it could be that global changes in circuit activity lead to synaptic abnormalities rather than vice versa. And there is some evidence of abnormalities occurring earlier in development, prior to synaptogenesis. For example, reduced neuron numbers (of cerebellar granule cells and cortical interneurons) have been observed during fetal development in humans, and in mouse models there are abnormalities in the timing of neuronal cell birth in the cortex, and in the development of thalamocortical axons. Hence, it will be important to determine the precise sequence of developmental abnormalities that occur in this syndrome.

RECOMMENDATIONS:
1. Undertake a systematic analysis of the development of key structures in the brains of people with Down syndrome using standardized techniques and measurements.

2. Understand the sequence of developmental events leading to the abnormal spine phenotype in mouse models of Down syndrome, and pursue the underlying genetic and cellular mechanisms.

3. Deploy studies in additional organisms such as C. elegans and Drosophila in which individual chromosome 21 genes can be perturbed, and the effects on the differentiation and maturation of individual neurons and synapses readily studied.

Protein, RNA, and Vesicle Trafficking

A wealth of information is now available concerning the mechanisms and molecules involved in synaptic vesicle trafficking at the synapse. Several key molecules involved in this process lie on chromosome 21, suggesting plausible hypotheses about how gene dosage might cause deficits in trafficking, spine morphology, and synaptic transmission. Moreover, enlarged endosomes constitute one of the earliest pathological hallmarks of Down syndrome in humans (appearing at 28 weeks of gestation); they are also seen in the *Ts65Dn* mouse model of Down syndrome. However, there is currently little information concerning the level of expression and activity of trafficking proteins in human Down syndrome tissue or mouse models, nor functional measures of trafficking in either case.

Because many of its component proteins are known, the synaptic vesicle trafficking system is a good candidate focus system for analyzing the functional impact of chromosome triplication on a specific biological output. This system would also allow one to analyze how the overexpression of a particular gene affects the expression of other genes within the same molecular pathway.

RECOMMENDATIONS:
1. Develop direct tests of the hypothesis that synaptic vesicle trafficking is disrupted in Down syndrome, including the use of banked human cells and mouse models.

2. Extend the analysis to an assessment of endocytosis and endosomal trafficking, again using both human and mouse tissues.

3. Develop panels of mice (or other model organisms) in which genes on chromosome 21, whose proteins are involved in vesicle trafficking and endocytosis, are systematically overexpressed, and analyze effects on trafficking, synaptic function, and the expression of other trafficking proteins.

Synapse Function

It seems highly likely that the neurophysiological, neuroanatomical, and cognitive deficits seen in Down syndrome are accompanied (if not caused by) defects in transmission at individual synapses. Interestingly, studies in the *Ts65Dn* mouse have shown a defect in long-term potentiation (LTP) at hippocampal synapses. LTP in turn has been postulated to underlie memory formation, which is known to be impaired in Down syndrome. However, there is little direct evidence about the nature of the synaptic defects in human Down syndrome. Identifying specific synaptic dysfunctions in Down syndrome will be key to: (1) generating better mouse models; and (2) developing simple *in vitro* assay systems to test therapeutics.

Other major gap areas include the lack of a current consensus about what behavioral phenotypes one would want to see in a mouse model of Down syndrome in order to deem it a "good" model. In addition, nothing is currently known about what synaptic defects may exist in the *Ts65Dn* mouse outside of the hippocampus. Hence, it would desirable to do a systematic survey of other major brain areas to obtain a more global picture of synaptic function in these animals. (A key step toward this goal would be to develop standardized functional assay methods to enable comparison of results from different labs.) Finally, a major obstacle to further progress has been the difficulty in obtaining reasonable quantities of mice for experiments. The most widely used and best characterized mouse model for Down syndrome is the *Ts65Dn* line. This line is difficult to breed and expensive to obtain, with mice costing $250 a pair. The high cost of mice and the difficulty in accessing adequate numbers is limiting research progress.

RECOMMENDATIONS
1. Characterize cognitive deficits in current mouse models to determine which mouse models best mimic the human disease. This endeavor should include input from psychologists/psychiatrists familiar with behavioral and cognitive deficits in human Down syndrome.

2. Survey synaptic deficits in Down syndrome model mice and determine which ones appear most closely associated with specific cognitive deficits, and which would be best for genotype/phenotype and therapeutics screening purposes.

3. Make existing mouse models available in larger numbers and at reduced cost.

4. Generate additional model mice, and perform genotype/phenotype analyses for cognitive and synaptic abnormalities.

5. Develop standardized methods for testing synaptic and cognitive function in Down syndrome model mice.

APP Processing and Transport

Amyloid plaques (which contain Abeta, a fragment of the APP protein) are seen in the brains of patients with Down syndrome, and look identical to those in AD. A similar mechanism may direct the production and deposition of Abeta in Down syndrome and Alzheimer disease. Thus, therapeutics aimed at Alzheimer disease could well be effective in Down syndrome as well. Amyloid deposition in Alzheimer disease is known to be due to defects in APP processing and transport. APP processing defects are also likely to play a role in Down syndrome because both APP and one of its processing enzymes (BACE 2) are located on chromosome 21. Indeed, one can readily conceive of means by which misprocessing and/or mistrafficking of APP in Down syndrome recreates the pathological changes evident in Alzheimer disease. However, while the biochemistry of APP processing in Alzheimer disease has been studied extensively, relatively little is known about the details of APP biochemistry in Down syndrome or the consequences for neuronal function of overexpression and the possible misprocessing and mistrafficking of APP.

Mitochondrial dysfunction is believed to contribute to amyloid deposition in Alzheimer disease. Down syndrome patients and model mice exhibit defects in mitochondrial function, some of which have been directly demonstrated to cause abnormalities in APP processing similar to those seen in Down syndrome. Thus, improvement of mitochondrial function appears to be another key therapeutic goal.

RECOMMENDATIONS
1. Use amyloid imaging technique to analyze more carefully the earliest stages of amyloid plaque formation in patients with Down syndrome and establish more precisely the target time window for early therapeutics and further investigation of pathobiology.

2. Establish cellular locations of defects in APP processing and trafficking and the consequences of such defects for neuronal development and maintenance.

3. Investigate intensively the biochemistry of APP processing in humans with Down syndrome and in animal models, including mechanisms of APP trafficking and amyloid beta production, degradation, and clearance.

4. More fully describe the defects in mitochondrial function in Down syndrome, and begin developing targeted therapeutics in vitro or in mouse models.

5. Encourage the inclusion of patients with Down syndrome in clinical trials of potential Alzheimer disease therapeutics.

From Synapse to Cognition and Behavior

Studies of cognition in Down syndrome suggest selective impairment of functions subserved by the hippocampus, prefrontal cortex, and cerebellum. Of these, hippocampal functions appear most profoundly impaired, suggesting that the hippocampus would be a good focus area for future work correlating genetic, cellular, and behavioral deficits. Hippocampal functions that have been demonstrated to be impaired in Down syndrome include exploration, context learning, and spatial cognition. Paradoxically, specific measures and testing regimens for these domains have been developed and validated far more extensively in animal models than in humans, especially children.

A great deal of variability is seen in cognitive function among Down syndrome patients. Understanding the genetic and environmental factors underlying this variability could be critical to improving function for those individuals at the lower end of the spectrum. For example, educational measures seem a promising area. However, we currently know little (from the neuroscience and cognition perspectives) about how education operates on "normal" young minds, much less the minds of children with Down syndrome. Another gap is in understanding cognitive function and development in individuals with Down syndrome at very young ages, from birth to five years or so.

Finally, most mechanistic studies of Down syndrome have been oriented at exploring the cellular and molecular pathobiology based on known functions of chromosome 21 genes or anatomical abnormalities seen in humans. Another approach would be to do drug screening studies on cognitive function in animal models such as *Drosophila* or mouse, and let the results of those inform mechanistic studies.

RECOMMENDATIONS

1. Develop better measures of hippocampal function in humans with Down syndrome.

2. Develop cognitive batteries that could be used across the lifespan, and use them to explore the developmental and age-related progression of Down syndrome.

3. Link these observations with studies of cognition in mouse models of Down syndrome.

4. Distinguish region-specific versus global impairments in neural function.

5. Ascertain whether or not synaptic dysfunction is linked to abnormal cognition.

6. Connect cellular mechanisms and genetic factors to synaptic and cognitive phenotypes.

7. Explore the genetic and environmental determinants of variability of cognitive function in Down syndrome patients.

8. Develop collaborations with educators, neuropharmacologists, and members of the pharmaceutical industry to begin testing educational and pharmacological interventions.

Overall Recommendations

In addition to specific recommendations listed above, several key focus areas emerged that pertained across all topics:

1. Eliminate barriers to progress and communication

   - Establish an inter-Institute working group at NIH to define short- and long-term objectives for the field, identify infrastructure needs, and promote sharing of animal models and reagents.
   - Develop collaborations with educators and members of the pharmaceutical industry to explore potential interventions.
   - Raise the consciousness of the neuroscience community to Down syndrome as a research topic with the hope of attracting new investigators to field (for example, by developing a symposium at the Society for Neuroscience meeting).

2. Model development:

   - Carry out descriptive studies in parallel in humans and mice to define anatomical, synaptic, functional, and cognitive phenotypes over the lifespan, and understand how they are correlated.
   - Identify a few well-defined phenotypes to focus on for further study that can be clearly linked to cognitive deficits seen in human Down syndrome, and develop standardized assays for these. The hippocampus seems a reasonable area to focus on in this regard; human studies suggest that prefrontal cortex and cerebellum should also be explored further.
   - Develop standardized assays for synaptic and cognitive function in Down syndrome patients and animal models.

3. Resource development

   - Establish a national patient registry:
     o Well-characterized cohort of patients for genotype-phenotype investigations (~1000 patients)
     o Couple with DNA database
   - Establish a Down syndrome brain bank, cell line repository, and DNA repository.
   - Increase supply of old and new mouse models and of needed reagents (and promote sharing among new and established researchers).
   - Support database development.
   - Prepare for clinical trials of ongoing treatments.

APPENDIX D: SUMMARY OF RESPONSES TO COMMENTS RECEIVED

The NIH received more than 150 comments on its draft *Research Plan for Down Syndrome* during the open comment period; responses came from families of individuals with Down syndrome and others in their communities, and from researchers across the country. The majority of respondents agreed with the Working Group that a plan is critical to promoting and advancing research on the wide range of possible issues related to Down syndrome.

In addition, a number of specific comments raised were carefully considered by the Working Group. Most of these comments were grouped according to subject and were addressed as described below.

INCREASE SCIENTIFIC AND OTHER COLLABORATIONS

The Working Group is aware that collaborative efforts on behalf of Down syndrome research are already occurring and agrees that the NIH needs to further expand its involvement in such efforts. In addition, some international collaborations were described during recent scientific meetings, and participation in these efforts might reduce the need for additional infrastructure. Consequently, the Working Group has expanded several of the research objectives in the final plan to reflect these interests.

INCREASE THE PACE OF RESEARCH

A number of comments included requests that the NIH proceed rapidly on the research objectives, and that some of the objectives be moved into the "short-term" category. While the Working Group shares the view that the NIH research portfolio on Down syndrome and related topics needs to be rebuilt, it will take some time to accomplish these objectives, partly due to the process for encouraging additional applications and scientific review. The Working Group agreed that the timeframes set forth in the plan are realistic, even ambitious, but will work diligently to meet them.

INCREASE FUNDING FOR RESEARCH ON DOWN SYNDROME

In its annual appropriations for the NIH, Congress does not earmark funds for specific diseases or conditions. Consequently, in implementing the *NIH Research Plan for Down Syndrome*, the NIH's focus will be on maximizing funds that are currently available by expanding collaborations so funds can be spent in the most cost-effective manner possible, and by working to ensure that researchers can utilize all available animal models and other scientific resources at the lowest possible cost. In addition, NIH program staff will continue to encourage high-quality investigator-initiated grant applications to increase the proportion of research focused on Down syndrome.

CREATE BOTH A CENTRAL DATABASE AND REGISTRY FOR DOWN SYNDROME

The Working Group agrees that a central database would provide a useful resource for researchers nationwide. Language has been added to the research objectives to reflect the Group's intent to move forward in creating or expanding a database, first reviewing current models and following the progress of the database proposed by the European Union; if appropriate, NIH will consider collaborating with one or more of these models to reduce duplicative efforts.

Regarding the registry, the NIH is aware that the Centers for Disease Control and Prevention (CDC) has established a prototype registry and does not want to duplicate those efforts. The Working Group will follow up with the CDC and share expertise as appropriate.

EXPAND OR CREATE A TISSUE BANK

A tissue bank that would meet the needs of researchers who wish to do research related to Down syndrome is a critically important resource. Language strengthening the research objective related to the tissue bank has been added to the plan.

AVAILABILITY OF TRISOMIC MICE AS ANIMAL MODELS

Echoing points raised by many in the research community during several scientific meetings, the NIH is already exploring ways to make increased numbers of mouse models available to funded researchers during the recompetition of the contract in fiscal year 2008.

EXPAND INFORMATION/COMMUNICATIONS ON DOWN SYNDROME

Numerous comments suggested the creation of a NIH Down syndrome Web site including information for parents and families of individuals with Down syndrome, clinicians, and researchers. In response, a new objective has been added to the plan (see the *Living with Down Syndrome* section); NIH will review other condition-specific pages currently available on its Web site and will create a new page for Down syndrome.

DEVELOP GUIDELINES REGARDING PRENATAL DIAGNOSIS

The NIH does not develop or publish practice guidelines for the medical/health professions. However, research results are shared with the medical community in several ways to inform the development or refinement of guidelines. In addition to articles in professional journals and other publications, NIH staff frequently attend and present at national meetings and conferences. Additional information on NIH-supported research will be provided on the new Web page.

CONDUCT RESEARCH ON INTRAUTERINE INTERVENTIONS

At this time, there is no evidence base of research (animal studies) on valid intrauterine interventions that could improve cognition or motor skills in individuals with Down syndrome. NIH staff will remain alert for investigator-initiated applications in this area.

ESTABLISH STANDARD BATTERY OF COGNITIVE TESTS FOR USE IN RESEARCH

Many cognitive tests have been developed to answer a narrow set of questions, but these are not appropriate for measuring an entire population or age group. NIH staff will review current grants and determine how results may be applied to different populations, with particular attention to whether these findings can be applied to translational research in which individuals with Down syndrome may be participating.

ADD OBJECTIVES REGARDING RESEARCH ON THE DEVELOPMENT OF MOTOR SKILLS IN PERSONS WITH DOWN SYNDROME

NIH funded a range of research on the development of motor skills two decades ago, but these efforts were not specific to Down syndrome. Language has been added to two research objectives to reflect a commitment to review that literature and to explore how research results may be moved into translation for individuals with Down syndrome, and if necessary, renew calls for such research.

CONDUCT RESEARCH ON OTHER COMORBID CONDITIONS

Several comments requested that the research objective listing comorbid conditions for Down syndrome be expanded so that it is clear that research in these areas is welcome; the objective has been expanded.

REFER SPECIFICALLY TO MEMANTINE AND OTHER THERAPEUTIC AGENTS IN DESCRIBING CLINICAL TRIALS

NIH cannot appear to endorse specific compounds; the research objectives are intentionally broadly stated to encompass therapies being used in current clinical trials.

ADD OBJECTIVE ON THE USE OF STATINS

Currently, NIH is not aware of a formal research study of statins in young people with Down syndrome. However, investigator-initiated applications in this area are encouraged.

ESTABLISH A STANDING COMMITTEE OF NON-NIH SCIENTISTS AND OTHERS TO MANAGE THE NIH DOWN SYNDROME RESEARCH PORTFOLIO; AND DESIGNATE A "CHAMPION" WITHIN THE NIH FOR RESEARCH ON DOWN SYNDROME

The NIH Director, acting through the NICHD, has established the trans-NIH Down Syndrome Working Group, which comprises the lead scientific staff from several Institutes and Centers in this area and others. The Working Group plans to continue to meet regularly to implement this research plan, and is committed to consulting frequently with non-NIH scientists and organizations representing the interests of individuals with Down syndrome and their families for input on future funding opportunities and related research efforts.

APPENDIX E. A SHORT HISTORY OF DOWN SYNDROME RESEARCH AND THE ROLE OF THE NIH

Two descriptions of some of the features associated with Down syndrome appear in the writings of physicians before the 1850s (Esquirol, 1838; Seguin, 1846). However, it was only after a systematic association of a number of consistent clinical features in a population of individuals in an asylum in England, that John Langdon Down provided the first classification of the clinical entity now recognized as Down syndrome in 1866. In 1876, two physicians attending a wealthy gentleman in his mid-20s noted that the patient seemed to exhibit premature aging (baldness, lack of skin tone, etc.) and the other features of the condition that Dr. Down described, christening the "syndrome described by Dr. Down" as a distinct clinical entity.

Because of demand for education by wealthy families in Europe for their intellectually disabled children, Montessori developed her now classical teaching methods in the 1880s. This approach, however, had little impact on the many individuals consigned often from birth to asylums for the insane and mentally unfit throughout Europe. Individuals with Down syndrome who survived infancy and childhood in such environments were often mistaken for cretins. Sutherland in 1900, however, demonstrated that while cretins responded to supplementation by thyroid extract, individuals with Down syndrome often did not. This was but the first of a series of endocrinologic abnormalities clinicians would come to associate with Down syndrome over the next century.

Life expectancy for individuals with Down syndrome remained very poor through the first decades of the new century. Physicians encouraged most parents to surrender their children who survived the perinatal period to state institutions. In such institutions, the high incidence of congenital heart disease, the compromised immune function, the increased frequency of childhood cancers, and the intellectual developmental delay made survival past the first decade rare.

Many investigators who examined and studied individuals with Down syndrome through the first seven decades of the twentieth century, as a result, did so in association with or as the staff of such institutions, where they elucidated many of the neurological consequences, anatomically, physiologically, and biochemically. In 1929, Struwe described the pathological features of the brain and noted that, at the cellular level, the brains of individuals with Down syndrome were very similar to those described by Alzheimer in a 54- year-old woman in 1906. However, those pathological features were apparent decades earlier in Down syndrome individuals, consistent with the prevailing notion of premature aging in that population.

Other features consistently associated with Down syndrome also became apparent during the 1920s and 1930s. Down syndrome individuals were often the youngest members of their birth family and advancing maternal age, as a result, often associated with the incidence of Down syndrome. Further, because the features of Down syndrome made it a recognizable condition throughout the world, there was increasing suspicion that the condition was "genetic." Examination of the prevalence of the condition, however, seemed to be relatively consistent among the world's ethnic groups, at about 1 in 800 to 1,000 live births.

With the discovery of antibiotics in the 1940s and the move to more structured state residential facilities for the intellectually disabled, the survival of some Down syndrome populations around the United States began to improve. Life expectancy in the 1950s had increased to about 15 years for those individuals who did not have congenital heart disease, succumb to infection, or develop cancer in childhood. Because most of the populations placed in institutions were Caucasian, it was not until the mid-1960s that the racial disparity in survival became very apparent, with few African Americans with Down syndrome surviving infancy. Life expectancy for African Americans with Down syndrome today is about 35 years, much less than the more than 50 year life expectancy of Caucasians with Down syndrome.

During the 1930s through the 1960s investigators characterized many of the neurochemical features associated with Down syndrome brains. They established the compromised function of many different cell populations, which affected many different neurotransmitter systems: noradrenergic, serotoninergic, cholinergic, and GABAergic. It was not until the 1970s that they established the full complement of neurochemical effects with the revelation that Down syndrome also affected peptidergic and amino acid transmitter systems, as well as many neurotrophic factors. Thus, there appears to be no neurotransmitter system spared compromise in the Down syndrome brain. In addition to decreases in the level of specific neurotransmitters, there are effects on neurotransmitter receptors, their structure, and function.

In 1959, two groups published the chromosomal basis of Down syndrome, triplication of human chromosome 21, and thus, established its true genetic basis. Improvements in cytogenetic techniques over the next 10 years, established clearly that although 95 percent of individuals with Down syndrome had triplication of the entire 21st chromosome, about 1 percent to 2 percent had only a part of the chromosome triplicated, and the remaining 4 percent had a part of the extra chromosome attached to another chromosome. Increasingly, geneticists began to pay attention to the similarities and differences among the characteristic features of each of the groups of individuals. This enabled them to make correlations, particularly in partially trisomic individuals, with specific phenotypic characteristics that commonly occurred when specific genes or clusters of genes were in triplicate.

In the early 1960s, legislation establishing the NICHD was quickly followed by a formal reorganization of the new Institute, approved by the Surgeon General, that named mental retardation and related research as one of NICHD's four main research priorities. Investigators established a number of these centers in locations with substantial residential populations of intellectually disabled individuals. This drew many investigators who previously confined their studies to other clinical conditions or to typically developing populations to the study of individuals with intellectual disabilities. Because the NIH through the NICHD provided these centers approximately $1 million per year to support for research with minimal intervention until 1988, many investigators studied Down syndrome as affiliates of these centers, but not necessarily as NIH grantees. Increasingly, other investigators began to characterize the features of Down syndrome that affect various organ systems, cardiovascular, gastrointestinal, immune, etc. They established that a number of features of Down syndrome do not occur typically in other genetic conditions, and increasingly sought to correlate the association of those features with specific genes or clusters of genes present on chromosome 21.

In the early 1960s, researchers turned increasingly to cellular characterization of specific cell populations. For example, immunologists recognized the exquisite sensitivity of Down syndrome cells to exposure to interferon. Oncologists began to recognize that specific childhood cancers such as megakaryoblastic leukemias were more common among the leukemias in Down syndrome children. Cardiologists documented the failure of endocardial cushion cells in the heart to complete the formation of the atrioventricular septum and the valves. Gastroenterologists established the failure of portions of the small intestine to reestablish a lumen, often in association with malrotation of the intestines. Because Down syndrome children were often born with substantial birth defects that were life threatening in the immediate perinatal period, clinicians and ethicists debated openly whether clinicians should provide any medical or surgical intervention and such treatment often did not occur.

Some investigators studying the nervous system used the Golgi method to reveal altered dendritic spine formation and architecture in cortical and hippocampal pyramidal cells. Other investigators determined that such changes were present in very young individuals with Down syndrome and that some changes were even present in fetal life. Still others focused on developmental trajectories and found that although there was developmental delay, for many of the specimens examined, the rate of development was parallel. Electrophysiologists with access to postmortem tissue began the first exploration of the physiological characteristics of neurons derived from both the central and peripheral nervous system of Down syndrome individuals. Still others documented the reduction of specific cell populations throughout the brain.

During the 1970s, many residential state institutions ceased to admit individuals with intellectual and developmental disabilities. As a consequence, more and more children remained with their birth families. Others were placed in adoptive homes. That dramatic social change produced two lasting effects. The first effect was that families now became increasingly invested in the medical care of children with Down syndrome and more parents pursued medical and surgical intervention for birth defects associated with Down syndrome. Further, parents increasingly required educational institutions to provide an inclusive learning environment to previously excluded populations. Such inclusion provided a venue for much research into the developmental trajectories, strengths, and weaknesses in cognitive development that individuals with Down syndrome experienced. Many psychologists and educators began to focus studies that involved the participation of children with Down syndrome at various levels, the family, the school, and the community.

Not only did the investigators study the characteristics of cognitive function and the nature of the intellectual disability, but they also began to examine the dynamics of family life, the choice to adopt and rear a disabled child, and the consequences of increasing social interaction and involvement of individuals with Down syndrome throughout the lifespan.

Psychologists found, as had many other investigators studying Down syndrome, that although most individuals could agree that the physical features of Down syndrome enabled its common recognition, Down syndrome individuals exhibited quite a remarkable variability in cognitive capacity and in developmental milestone attainment. For example, some children with Down syndrome spoke their first sentence at age one, whereas others did so at age seven and some never did. As a consequence of basic research that demonstrated altered brain function in animals placed in enriched environments, the next decade of research involved studies of the effects of early and later infant stimulation, its duration, and its intensity. Intensive efforts to improve speech and communication skills led investigators to focus on differences in auditory and visual learning and to design methods to facilitate the relative "strengths" of individual children.

A study published in 1979 described the impact of stimulation on Down syndrome infants and children. Children with Down syndrome raised in institutions had an average IQ of 20 to 30. Those raised at home with no specific attention to stimulation averaged about 40, and those raised at home with stimulation had an average of 55. This study also found that IQ declines with age in people with Down syndrome, regardless of their environment.

Paralleling this increased interest in behavioral and biobehavioral aspects of the development of Down syndrome came rapid strides in the ability to identify the specific genes located on individual human chromosomes. In 1973, investigators localized the first two of many genes to human chromosome 21. Other investigators focused on the genomes of other mammals: mouse, dog, cat, sheep, goat, cow, and horse. From such comparative genetic studies emerged the concept that the cluster of genes located on human chromosome 21 often had remained together and in the same order since the divergence of mice and men 60 million years ago. This led investigators in the 1980s to increasingly make comparisons of the genes shared among the various mammalian chromosomes.

The development of the first animal models of aneuploidy in the mid-1970s helped further such investigation. Noting the unusual arrangement of chromosomes in the mice that populated the Poschiavinus valley in the Alps (*Mus poschiavinus*, the tobacco mouse), Alfred Gropp came upon a strategy to create aneuploidy for each of the 19 mouse chromosomes. His use of such Robertsonian translocation stocks to generate trisomy led the NICHD to fund its first contract to characterize and ultimately distribute such stocks to investigators in the late 1970s. Based solely on his pathological characterization, Gropp concluded that fetal mice with trisomy 16 most closely resembled Down syndrome fetuses. Many developed fetal hydrops (nuchal translucency), had congenital heart disease affecting the atrioventricular septum and valves, had poor liver and endocrine organ development, had similar facial features, and like many fetuses with Down syndrome, died *in utero*. As genes localized to human chromosome 21 also clustered to mouse chromosome 16, there was significant interest in the research community to study these mice. Unfortunately, since much brain development in mice occurs postnatally, investigators needed a "better mouse model."

Even given the limitations of the trisomy 16 mouse model, a number of groups of investigators competed successfully for NIH funds during the 1980s in the form of individual research grants, program project grants, and contracts to study and characterize the trisomy 16 mouse. Important to the validity of that mouse as a model for studies relevant to Down syndrome and before the substantial comparative genetic mapping effort, was characterization of these mice, and other mice with trisomy of other chromosomes, at the structural, physiological, and biochemical levels. During the 1970s and 1980s, there was substantial concern in the research community that it was not so much the particular genes in triplicate, but the amount of genetic material in triplicate that was source of the phenotypic features observed. Since chromosome 21 is the smallest human autosome, it was natural for investigators to focus studies on chromosome 19 in the mouse. Structurally, developmentally, and neurochemically, the trisomy 19 mouse differed from individuals with Down syndrome, but served as a very useful comparison organism. With further study and characterization, the trisomy 16 mouse emerged as the mouse trisomy that resembled the Down syndrome phenotype most closely.

With more detailed genetic examination of mouse chromosome 16, it became clear to investigators that mouse chromosome 16 was not an exact ortholog to human chromosome 21. Rather, its long arm contained genes for only a portion of human chromosome 21 and the rest of the genes located on human chromosome 21 were primarily located on two other mouse chromosomes, 10 and 17. This led investigators to attempt to develop other mouse models that more closely resembled Down syndrome genetically.

By the late 1980s the contract to supply Robertsonian translocation stocks moved to the Jackson Laboratory and another contract to generate mice with partial trisomy of various chromosomes enabled Muriel Davisson to generate a mouse with triplication of many of the genes human chromosome 21 and mouse chromosome 16 share, the *Ts65Dn* mouse. Although the males, like most Down syndrome males, were sterile, investigators could breed the females through elaborative and intensive husbandry to generate litters that contained the partially trisomic mice. Because these mice had a more modest phenotype, they required elaborate genetic characterization that few laboratories could conduct. These mice were viable into adult life and enabled much intensive investigation of the similarities and differences that occurred in various organ systems.

During the 1980s investigators began to direct studies to the basis of aneuploidy in human populations. Epidemiologic and genetic studies increasingly focused on the source of the extra chromosome, the timing of its generation, and factors that affect the frequency of aneuploidy. Although it was generally accepted that women who were older than age 35 were at much greater risk for having a child with Down syndrome (1:60), most Down syndrome children are born to women younger than age 35, where the risk is much less. Further, very frequently the source of the extra chromosome is the mother and the timing of its generation during meiosis varies with maternal age. Investigators studying fetal ovaries found that some errors in meiosis occurred as early as the fifth month of gestation (when the mother was a fetus), while general population studies found that other errors occurred during the preparation of the egg for ovulation during the mother's reproductive life.

With further development of the comparative genetics of mouse and human and increased emphasis on the study of the genetics of Alzheimer disease in the 1980s, investigators placed greater focus on specific genes present on human chromosome 21 and the relation of their overexpression to the pathological characteristics of Alzheimer disease and other neurologic conditions. Generation of mice with specific mouse or human transgenes enabled investigators to dissect further the contributions of specific genes to the overall phenotype observed. Although it was well accepted that individuals with Down syndrome develop the neuropathologic characteristics of Alzheimer disease as many as 50 years earlier, it was not until a longitudinal cohort study began to examine the aging process in Down syndrome that the similarities and differences began to emerge. Now well into its second decade of funding, this program project continues to collect substantial data on a cohort of individuals, their medical care, their medical issues, and the characteristics that predispose some of them to the development of dementia as they age.

With the development of amniocentesis in the 1970s and of chorionic villus biopsy in the 1980s, it became possible for clinicians to offer prenatal diagnosis for a variety of genetic conditions. With more women choosing to delay childbearing until their fourth or fifth decade of life, many more of these older women were at substantial risk for a pregnancy with an aneuploid embryo or fetus. Because pregnancies involving an embryo or fetus with aneuploidy frequently end in spontaneous loss or stillbirth, several groups of investigators began to focus on the best methods to detect aneuploid conception at earlier gestational ages. This led not only to population studies that compared the rate of detection, but also the accuracy of detection at various gestational ages. Other studies examined whether non-invasive detection could enable reliable detection of aneuploid cells in maternal blood.

The 1990s was a decade of intense research focus on the brain, its development, and its function. Increasing numbers of investigators were drawn to Down syndrome research through program solicitations with focus on specific aspects of Down syndrome, such as cognitive function. In addition, behavioral and biobehavioral investigators amassed during the previous decade considerable information on Down syndrome individuals compared with other individuals with intellectual and developmental disabilities. With the efforts of the Human Genome Project to map the entire human genome, more and more genes came to associate with specific conditions. Down syndrome individuals became the most common intellectually disabled comparison group in the studies of many investigators.

A number of investigators developed models in mice and other organisms to study more directly the cellular and molecular consequences of triplication of genes located on human chromosome 21. Other partial trisomies in mice, such as *Ts1Cje*, triplicated a smaller region of mouse chromosome 16 and enabled investigators to examine more closely the neurobiologic consequences of triplication of specific clusters of genes. Studies using other organisms, such as *Drosophila*, enabled investigators to examine the consequences of triplication of specific genes on developmental processes in a much shorter time frame. Studies of non-human primates enabled examination of expression of specific genes, both spatially and temporally.

Because of the dramatic increase in life expectancy of individuals with Down syndrome, nearly tripling since the 1970s, researchers also began to focus attention increasingly from children with Down syndrome to adults and increasingly to elderly individuals with Down syndrome. Behavioral and biobehavioral investigators directed focus on the family dynamics of transition from childhood to adult, acquisition of skills applicable to both workplace and independent living, issues of aging caregivers and sibling relationships, and the transition during the elder period to nursing home care. With the increased risk of Alzheimer dementia in elderly individuals with Down syndrome, several clinical trials examined the effects of various medications and antioxidant combinations on the development of dementia or its progress. Others conducted limited and focused trials of specific medications in children, but often studied too few individuals to derive concrete and meaningful results. Long-term longitudinal studies enabled investigators to follow medical histories and the use of various common medications among Down syndrome individuals and to provide insight into whether or not they age atypically.

In 2000, a consortium of researchers published the DNA sequence of the whole of human chromosome 21, followed several years later by another consortium's publication of the complete sequence of mouse chromosome 16. With completion of the sequences for other mouse and human chromosomes, investigators could continue to develop mouse models for Down syndrome research. Currently, investigators have developed a number of such partial trisomies, including *Ts1Rhr*, *Ts2Cje*, *Ts1Yu*, and a mouse containing portions of human chromosome 21 as an episome, Tc1.

Behavioral and biobehavioral investigators have begun to partner with basic researchers to conduct multidisciplinary studies of populations of Down syndrome individuals. In addition to longitudinal cognitive assessments, investigators have applied evoked response potential electrophysiology and magnetoencephalography to very young children and have found that the "signatures" of the ERP profile often are distinctive for a given intellectual and developmental disability. These signatures mature rapidly over time and may predict subsequent cognitive capability during early childhood. Still other investigators use functional imaging techniques on older individuals with Down syndrome and positron emission tomography to reveal changes in metabolic function within the brain during the aging process.

Interested readers can find many of the results of research of the past decade in the summary reports of various meeting sponsored by the NIH over the past several years, including a meeting on cognitive function in Down syndrome, the Gatlinburg Conference of 2007, and an experts meeting to advise the NIH Down Syndrome Working Group.

APPENDIX F. NIH-SUPPORTED DOWN SYNDROME RESEARCH: A SELECTED BIBLIOGRAPHY

The following citations resulted from a search of MEDLINE, the premier biomedical literature database of the National Library of Medicine, using the following: Down syndrome [keyword], Research Support, N.I.H. [keyword], and Extramural [publication type].

The keyword [Research Support, N.I.H.] is a designation for publications of research resulting from extramural research funded by the National Institutes of Health. This keyword was introduced in 2005.

2007

Hattori D, Demir E, Kim HW, Viragh E, Zipursky SL, & Dickson BJ. (2007). Dscam diversity is essential for neuronal wiring and self-recognition. *Nature, 449*, 223-227.

Orsmond GI, & Seltzer MM. (2007). Siblings of individuals with autism or Down syndrome: Effects on adult lives. *J Intellect Disabil Res, 51*, 682-696.

Breathnach FM, Malone FD, Lambert-Messerlian G, Cuckle HS, Porter TF, et al. (2007). First- and second-trimester screening: Detection of aneuploidies other than Down syndrome. *Obstet Gynecol, 110*, 651-657.

Cornish K, Scerif G, & Karmiloff-Smith A. (2007). Tracing syndrome-specific trajectories of attention across the lifespan. *Cortex, 43*, 672-685.

Sethupathy P, Borel C, Gagnebin M, Grant GR, Deutsch S, et al. (2007). Human microRNA-155 on chromosome 21 differentially interacts with its polymorphic target in the *AGTR1* 3' untranslated region: A mechanism for functional single-nucleotide polymorphisms related to phenotypes. *Am J Hum Genet, 81*, 405-413.

Prandini P, Deutsch S, Lyle R, Gagnebin M, Delucinge Vivier C, et al. (2007). Natural gene-expression variation in Down syndrome modulates the outcome of gene-dosage imbalance. *Am J Hum Genet, 81*, 252-263.

Belichenko PV, Kleschevnikov AM, Salehi A, Epstein CJ, & Mobley WC. (2007). Synaptic and cognitive abnormalities in mouse models of Down syndrome: Exploring genotype-phenotype relationships. *J Comp Neurol, 504*, 329-345.

Schupf N, Patel B, Pang D, Zigman WB, Silverman W, et al. (2007). Elevated plasma beta-amyloid peptide Abeta(42) levels, incident dementia, and mortality in Down syndrome. *Arch Neurol, 64*, 1007-1013.

Laifenfeld D, Patzek LJ, McPhie DL, Chen Y, Levites Y, et al. (2007). Rab5 mediates an amyloid precursor protein signaling pathway that leads to apoptosis. *J Neurosci, 27*, 7141-7153.

Gollogly LK, Ryeom SW, & Yoon SS. (2007). Down syndrome candidate region 1-like 1 (DSCR1-L1) mimics the inhibitory effects of DSCR1 on calcineurin signaling in endothelial cells and inhibits angiogenesis. *J Surg Res, 142,* 129-136.

Ball RH, Caughey AB, Malone FD, Nyberg DA, Comstock CH, et al. (2007). First- and second-trimester evaluation of risk for Down syndrome. *Obstet Gynecol, 110,* 10-17.

Bearer EL, Zhang X, & Jacobs RE. (2007). Live imaging of neuronal connections by magnetic resonance: Robust transport in the hippocampal-septal memory circuit in a mouse model of Down syndrome. *Neuroimage, 37,* 230-242.

Fernandez F, & Garner CC. (2007). Object recognition memory is conserved in *Ts1Cje*, a mouse model of Down syndrome. *Neurosci Lett, 421,* 137-141.

Bush CR, Havens JM, Necela BM, Su W, Chen L, et al. (2007). Functional genomic analysis reveals cross-talk between peroxisome proliferator-activated receptor gamma and calcium signaling in human colorectal cancer cells. *J Biol Chem, 282,* 23387-23401.

Dykens EM, & Hodapp RM. (2007). Three steps toward improving the measurement of behavior in behavioral phenotype research. *Child Adolesc Psychiatr Clin N Am, 16,* 617-630.

Keller-Bell YD, & Abbeduto LD. (2007). Narrative development in adolescents and young adults with fragile x syndrome. *Am J Ment Retard, 112,* 289-299.

Urbano RC, & Hodapp RM. (2007). Divorce in families of children with Down syndrome: A population-based study. *Am J Ment Retard, 112,* 261-274.

Roberts J, Price J, Barnes E, Nelson L, Burchinal M, et al. (2007). Receptive vocabulary, expressive vocabulary, and speech production of boys with fragile X syndrome in comparison to boys with Down syndrome. *Am J Ment Retard, 112,* 177-193.

Spiridigliozzi GA, Heller JH, Crissman BG, Sullivan-Saarela JA, Eells R, et al. (2007). Preliminary study of the safety and efficacy of donepezil hydrochloride in children with Down syndrome: A clinical report series. *Am J Med Genet A, 143,* 1408-1413.

Adayev T, Chen-Hwang MC, Murakami N, Lee E, Bolton DC, & Hwang YW. (2007). Dual-specificity tyrosine phosphorylation-regulated kinase 1A does not require tyrosine phosphorylation for activity *in vitro. Biochemistry, 46,* 7614-7624.

Sultan M, Piccini I, Balzereit D, Herwig R, Saran NG, et al. (2007). Gene expression variation in Down's syndrome mice allows prioritization of candidate genes. *Genome Biol, 8,* R91.

Parsons T, Ryan TM, Reeves RH, & Richtsmeier JT. (2007). Microstructure of trabecular bone in a mouse model for Down syndrome. *Anat Rec (Hoboken), 290,* 414-421.

Roberts J, Martin GE, Moskowitz L, Harris AA, Foreman J, & Nelson L. (2007). Discourse skills of boys with fragile X syndrome in comparison to boys with Down syndrome. *J Speech Lang Hear Res, 50,* 475-492.

Keller-Bell Y, & Fox RA. (2007). A preliminary study of speech discrimination in youth with Down syndrome. *Clin Linguist Phon, 21*, 305-317.

Bunn L, Roy EA, & Elliott D. (2007). Speech perception and motor control in children with Down syndrome. *Child Neuropsychol, 13*, 262-275.

Smith BA, Kubo M, Black DP, Holt KG, & Ulrich BD. (2007). Effect of practice on a novel task--walking on a treadmill: Preadolescents with and without Down syndrome. *Phys Ther, 87*, 766-777.

Aldridge K, Reeves RH, Olson LE, & Richtsmeier JT. (2007). Differential effects of trisomy on brain shape and volume in related aneuploid mouse models. *Am J Med Genet A, 143*, 1060-1070.

Busciglio J, Pelsman A, Helguera P, Ashur-Fabian O, Pinhasov A, et al. (2007). NAP and ADNF-9 protect normal and Down's syndrome cortical neurons from oxidative damage and apoptosis. *Curr Pharm Des, 13*, 1091-1098.

Hill CA, Reeves RH, & Richtsmeier JT. (2007). Effects of aneuploidy on skull growth in a mouse model of Down syndrome. *J Anat, 210*, 394-405.

Li Z, Yu T, Morishima M, Pao A, LaDuca J, et al. (2007). Duplication of the entire 22.9 Mb human chromosome 21 syntenic region on mouse chromosome 16 causes cardiovascular and gastrointestinal abnormalities. *Hum Mol Genet, 16*, 1359-1366.

Visootsak J, & Sherman S. (2007). Neuropsychiatric and behavioral aspects of trisomy 21. *Curr Psychiatry Rep, 9*, 135-140.

Van Riper M. (2007). Families of children with Down syndrome: Responding to "a change in plans" with resilience. *J Pediatr Nurs, 22*, 116-128.

Nagalla SR, Canick JA, Jacob T, Schneider KA, Reddy AP, et al. (2007). Proteomic analysis of maternal serum in Down syndrome: Identification of novel protein biomarkers. *J Proteome Res, 6*, 1245-1257.

Risinger JI, Chandramouli GV, Maxwell GL, Custer M, Pack S, et al. (2007). Global expression analysis of cancer/testis genes in uterine cancers reveals a high incidence of BORIS expression. *Clin Cancer Res, 13*, 1713-1719.

Head E, Lott IT, Patterson D, Doran E, & Haier RJ. (2007). Possible compensatory events in adult Down syndrome brain prior to the development of Alzheimer disease neuropathology: Targets for nonpharmacological intervention. *J Alzheimers Dis, 11*, 61-76.

Zigman WB, Schupf N, Jenkins EC, Urv TK, Tycko B, & Silverman W. (2007). Cholesterol level, statin use and Alzheimer's disease in adults with Down syndrome. *Neurosci Lett, 416*, 279-284.

Olson LE, Roper RJ, Sengstaken CL, Peterson EA, Aquino V, et al. (2007). Trisomy for the Down syndrome "critical region" is necessary but not sufficient for brain phenotypes of trisomic mice. *Hum Mol Genet, 16*, 774-782.

Xing L, Salas M, Lin CS, Zigman W, Silverman W, et al. (2007). Faithful tissue-specific expression of the human chromosome 21-linked *COL6A1* gene in BAC-transgenic mice. *Mamm Genome, 18*, 113-122.

Fidler DJ, Philofsky A, & Hepburn SL. (2007). Language phenotypes and intervention planning: Bridging research and practice. *Ment Retard Dev Disabil Res Rev, 13*, 47-57.

Roberts JE, Price J, & Malkin C. (2007). Language and communication development in Down syndrome. *Ment Retard Dev Disabil Res Rev, 13*, 26-35.

Fernandez F, Morishita W, Zuniga E, Nguyen J, Blank M, et al. (2007). Pharmacotherapy for cognitive impairment in a mouse model of Down syndrome. *Nat Neurosci, 10*, 411-413.

Yutzey KE, & Robbins J. (2007). Principles of genetic murine models for cardiac disease. *Circulation, 115*, 792-799.

Craig WY, Haddow JE, Palomaki GE, & Roberson M. (2007). Major fetal abnormalities associated with positive screening tests for Smith-Lemli-Opitz syndrome (SLOS). *Prenat Diagn, 27*, 409-414.

Mehta PD, Capone G, Jewell A, & Freedland RL. (2007). Increased amyloid beta protein levels in children and adolescents with Down syndrome. *J Neurol Sci, 254*, 22-27.

Wegiel J, Kuchna I, Nowicki K, Frackowiak J, Mazur-Kolecka B, et al. (2007). Intraneuronal Abeta immunoreactivity is not a predictor of brain amyloidosis-beta or neurofibrillary degeneration. *Acta Neuropathol (Berl), 113*, 389-402.

Ronan A, Fagan K, Christie L, Conroy J, Nowak NJ, & Turner G. (2007). Familial 4.3 Mb duplication of 21q22 sheds new light on the Down syndrome critical region. *J Med Genet, 44*, 448-451.

Freeman SB, Allen EG, Oxford-Wright CL, Tinker SW, Druschel C, et al. (2007). The National Down Syndrome Project: Design and implementation. *Public Health Rep, 122*, 62-72.

Vyas P, & Crispino JD. (2007). Molecular insights into Down syndrome-associated leukemia. *Curr Opin Pediatr, 19*, 9-14.

Ruser TF, Arin D, Dowd M, Putnam S, Winklosky B, et al. (2007). Communicative competence in parents of children with autism and parents of children with specific language impairment. *J Autism Dev Disord, 37*, 1323-1336.

Barbaric D, Alonzo TA, Gerbing RB, Meshinchi S, Heerema NA, et al. (2007). Minimally differentiated acute myeloid leukemia (FAB AML-M0) is associated with an adverse outcome in children: A report from the Children's Oncology Group, studies CCG-2891 and CCG-2961. *Blood, 109*, 2314-2321.

Hanson JE, Blank M, Valenzuela RA, Garner CC, & Madison DV. (2007). The functional nature of synaptic circuitry is altered in area CA3 of the hippocampus in a mouse model of Down's syndrome. *J Physiol, 579*, 53-67.

Caughey AB, Musci TJ, Belluomini J, Main D, Otto C, & Goldberg J. (2007). Nuchal translucency screening: How do women actually utilize the results? *Prenat Diagn, 27*, 119-123.

Lavenex P, Banta Lavenex P, & Amaral DG. (2007). Postnatal development of the primate hippocampal formation. *Dev Neurosci, 29*, 179-192.

Dowjat WK, Adayev T, Kuchna I, Nowicki K, Palminiello S, et al. (2007). Trisomy-driven overexpression of DYRK1A kinase in the brain of subjects with Down syndrome. *Neurosci Lett, 413*, 77-81.

Best TK, Siarey RJ, & Galdzicki Z. (2007). *Ts65Dn*, a mouse model of Down syndrome, exhibits increased GABAB-induced potassium current. *J Neurophysiol, 97*, 892-900.

Kovalevskaya G, Kakuma T, Schlatterer J, O'Connor JF. (2007). Hyperglycosylated HCG expression in pregnancy: Cellular origin and clinical applications. *Mol Cell Endocrinol, 260-262*, 237-243.

Gimenez-Llort L, Blazquez G, Canete T, Johansson B, Oddo S, et al. (2007). Modeling behavioral and neuronal symptoms of Alzheimer's disease in mice: a role for intraneuronal amyloid. *Neurosci Biobehav Rev, 31*, 125-147.

Carter JC, Capone GT, Gray RM, Cox CS, & Kaufmann WE. (2007). Autistic-spectrum disorders in Down syndrome: Further delineation and distinction from other behavioral abnormalities. *Am J Med Genet B Neuropsychiatr Genet, 144*, 87-94.

Nistor M, Don M, Parekh M, Sarsoza F, Goodus M, et al. (2007). Alpha- and beta-secretase activity as a function of age and beta-amyloid in Down syndrome and normal brain. *Neurobiol Aging, 28*, 1493-1506.

Kwak HI, Gustafson T, Metz RP, Laffin B, Schedin P, & Porter WW. (2007). Inhibition of breast cancer growth and invasion by single-minded 2s. *Carcinogenesis, 28*, 259-266.

2006

Sahir N, Brenneman DE, & Hill JM. (2006). Neonatal mice of the Down syndrome model, *Ts65Dn*, exhibit upregulated VIP measures and reduced responsiveness of cortical astrocytes to VIP stimulation. *J Mol Neurosci, 30*, 329-340.

Heller JH, Spiridigliozzi GA, Crissman BG, Sullivan JA, Eells RL, et al. (2006). Safety and efficacy of rivastigmine in adolescents with Down syndrome: A preliminary 20-week, open-label study. *J Child Adolesc Psychopharmacol, 16*, 755-765.

Lott IT, Head E, Doran E, & Busciglio J. (2006). Beta-amyloid, oxidative stress and down syndrome. *Curr Alzheimer Res, 3*, 521-528.

Qin L, Zhao D, Liu X, Nagy JA, Hoang MV, et al. (2006). Down syndrome candidate region 1 isoform 1 mediates angiogenesis through the calcineurin-NFAT pathway. *Mol Cancer Res, 4*, 811-820.

Caviedes P, Caviedes R, & Rapoport SI. (2006). Altered calcium currents in cultured sensory neurons of normal and trisomy 16 mouse fetuses, an animal model for human trisomy 21 (Down syndrome). *Biol Res, 39*, 471-481.

Sharp FR, Xu H, Lit L, Walker W, Apperson M, et al. (2006). The future of genomic profiling of neurological diseases using blood. *Arch Neurol, 63*, 1529-1536.

Lewis P, Abbeduto L, Murphy M, Richmond E, Giles N, et al. (2006). Psychological well-being of mothers of youth with fragile X syndrome: Syndrome specificity and within-syndrome variability. *J Intellect Disabil Res, 50*, 894-904.

Adayev T, Chen-Hwang MC, Murakami N, Wang R, & Hwang YW. (2006). MNB/DYRK1A phosphorylation regulates the interactions of synaptojanin 1 with endocytic accessory proteins. *Biochem Biophys Res Commun, 351*, 1060-1065.

Canick JA, Lambert-Messerlian GM, Palomaki GE, Neveux LM, Malone FD, et al. (2006). Comparison of serum markers in first-trimester down syndrome screening. *Obstet Gynecol, 108*, 1192-1199.

Eddleman KA, Malone FD, Sullivan L, Dukes K, Berkowitz RL, et al. (2006). Pregnancy loss rates after midtrimester amniocentesis. *Obstet Gynecol, 108*, 1067-1072.

Savasan S, Buck S, Raimondi SC, Becton DL, Weinstein H, et al. (2006). CD36 (thrombospondin receptor) expression in childhood acute megakaryoblastic leukemia: *In vitro* drug sensitivity and outcome. *Leuk Lymphoma, 47*, 2076-2083.

Whitlock JA.(2006). Down syndrome and acute lymphoblastic leukaemia. *Br J Haematol, 135*, 595-602.

Meijer WM, Werler MM, Louik C, Hernandez-Diaz S, de Jong-van den Berg LT, & Mitchell AA. (2006). Can folic acid protect against congenital heart defects in Down syndrome? *Birth Defects Res A Clin Mol Teratol, 76*, 714-717.

Camarata S, Yoder P, & Camarata M. (2006). Simultaneous treatment of grammatical and speech-comprehensibility deficits in children with Down syndrome. *Downs Syndr Res Pract, 11*, 9-17.

Gardiner K, & Costa AC. (2006). The proteins of human chromosome 21. *Am J Med Genet C Semin Med Genet, 142*, 196-205.

Dixon N, Kishnani PS, & Zimmerman S. (2006). Clinical manifestations of hematologic and oncologic disorders in patients with Down syndrome. *Am J Med Genet C Semin Med Genet, 142*, 149-157.

Maslen CL, Babcock D, Robinson SW, Bean LJ, Dooley KJ, et al. (2006). *CRELD1* mutations contribute to the occurrence of cardiac atrioventricular septal defects in Down syndrome. *Am J Med Genet A, 140*, 2501-2505.

Linabery AM, Olshan AF, Gamis AS, Smith FO, Heerema NA, et al. (2006). Exposure to medical test irradiation and acute leukemia among children with Down syndrome: A report from the Children's Oncology Group. *Pediatrics, 118*, e1499-e1508.

Dickson CA, Deutsch CK, Wang SS, & Dube WV. (2006). Matching-to-sample assessment of stimulus overselectivity in students with intellectual disabilities. *Am J Ment Retard, 111*, 447-453.

Carrasco J, Adlard P, Cotman C, Quintana A, Penkowa M, et al. (2006). Metallothionein-I and -III expression in animal models of Alzheimer disease. *Neuroscience, 143*, 911-922.

Adayev T, Chen-Hwang MC, Murakami N, Wegiel J, & Hwang YW. (2006). Kinetic properties of a MNB/DYRK1A mutant suitable for the elucidation of biochemical pathways. *Biochemistry, 45*, 12011-12019.

Ailey SH, Miller AM, Heller T, & Smith EV, Jr.(2006). Evaluating an interpersonal model of depression among adults with Down syndrome. *Res Theory Nurs Pract, 20*, 229-246.

Looper J, Wu J, Angulo Barroso R, Ulrich D, & Ulrich BD. (2006). Changes in step variability of new walkers with typical development and with Down syndrome. *J Mot Behav, 38*, 367-372.

Shrestha BR, Vitolo OV, Joshi P, Lordkipanidze T, Shelanski M, & Dunaevsky A. (2006). Amyloid beta peptide adversely affects spine number and motility in hippocampal neurons. *Mol Cell Neurosci, 33*, 274-282.

Kingsbury MA, Yung YC, Peterson SE, Westra JW, & Chun J. (2006). Aneuploidy in the normal and diseased brain. *Cell Mol Life Sci, 63*, 2626-2641.

Comstock CH, Malone FD, Ball RH, Nyberg DA, Saade GR, et al. (2006). Is there a nuchal translucency millimeter measurement above which there is no added benefit from first trimester serum screening? *Am J Obstet Gynecol, 195*, 843-847.

Antonarakis SE, & Epstein CJ. (2006). The challenge of Down syndrome. *Trends Mol Med, 12*, 473-479.

Schupf N, Winsten S, Patel B, Pang D, Ferin M, et al. (2006). Bioavailable estradiol and age at onset of Alzheimer's disease in postmenopausal women with Down syndrome. *Neurosci Lett, 406*, 298-302.

Tabaton M, & Gambetti P. (2006). Soluble amyloid-beta in the brain: The scarlet pimpernel. *J Alzheimers Dis, 9*, 127-132.

Barnes EF, Roberts J, Mirrett P, Sideris J, & Misenheimer J. (2006). A comparison of oral structure and oral-motor function in young males with fragile X syndrome and Down syndrome. *J Speech Lang Hear Res, 49*, 903-917.

Siarey RJ, Kline-Burgess A, Cho M, Balbo A, Best TK, et al. (2006). Altered signaling pathways underlying abnormal hippocampal synaptic plasticity in the *Ts65Dn* mouse model of Down syndrome. *J Neurochem, 98*, 1266-1277.

Shukkur EA, Shimohata A, Akagi T, Yu W, Yamaguchi M, et al. (2006). Mitochondrial dysfunction and tau hyperphosphorylation in *Ts1Cje*, a mouse model for Down syndrome. *Hum Mol Genet, 15*, 2752-2762.

Podvin D, Kuehn CM, Mueller BA, & Williams M. (2006). Maternal and birth characteristics in relation to childhood leukaemia. *Paediatr Perinat Epidemiol, 20*, 312-322.

Latash ML, & Anson JG. (2006). Synergies in health and disease: Relations to adaptive changes in motor coordination. *Phys Ther, 86*, 1151-1160.

Fidler DJ, Hepburn S, & Rogers S. (2006). Early learning and adaptive behaviour in toddlers with Down syndrome: Evidence for an emerging behavioural phenotype? *Downs Syndr Res Pract, 9*, 37-44.

Chapman RS. (2006). Language learning in Down syndrome: The speech and language profile compared to adolescents with cognitive impairment of unknown origin. *Downs Syndr Res Pract, 10*, 61-66.

Liu K, Solano I, Mann D, Lemere C, Mercken M, et al. (2006). Characterization of Abeta11-40/42 peptide deposition in Alzheimer's disease and young Down's syndrome brains: Implication of N-terminally truncated Abeta species in the pathogenesis of Alzheimer's disease. *Acta Neuropathol (Berl), 112*, 163-174.

Kwak YD, Brannen CL, Qu T, Kim HM, Dong X, et al. (2006). Amyloid precursor protein regulates differentiation of human neural stem cells. *Stem Cells Dev, 15,* 381-389.

Muntean AG, Ge Y, Taub JW, & Crispino JD. (2006). Transcription factor GATA-1 and Down syndrome leukemogenesis. *Leuk Lymphoma, 47,* 986-997.

Craig WY, Haddow JE, Palomaki GE, Kelley RI, Kratz LE, et al. (2006). Identifying Smith-Lemli-Opitz syndrome in conjunction with prenatal screening for Down syndrome. *Prenat Diagn, 26,* 842-849.

Lorenzi HA, & Reeves RH. (2006). Hippocampal hypocellularity in the *Ts65Dn* mouse originates early in development. *Brain Res, 1104,* 153-159.

Salehi A, Delcroix JD, Belichenko PV, Zhan K, Wu C, et al. (2006). Increased App expression in a mouse model of Down's syndrome disrupts NGF transport and causes cholinergic neuron degeneration. *Neuron, 51,* 29-42.

Ma'ayan A, Gardiner K, & Iyengar R. (2006). The cognitive phenotype of Down syndrome: Insights from intracellular network analysis. *NeuroRx, 3,* 396-406.

Fey ME, Warren SF, Brady N, Finestack LH, Bredin-Oja SL, et al. (2006). Early effects of responsivity education/prelinguistic milieu teaching for children with developmental delays and their parents. *J Speech Lang Hear Res, 49,* 526-547.

Harashima C, Jacobowitz DM, Stoffel M, Chakrabarti L, Haydar TF, et al. (2006). Elevated expression of the G-protein-activated inwardly rectifying potassium channel 2 (GIRK2) in cerebellar unipolar brush cells of a Down syndrome mouse model. *Cell Mol Neurobiol, 26,* 719-734.

Dong Y, Taylor HE, & Dimopoulos G. (2006). AgDscam, a hypervariable immunoglobulin domain-containing receptor of the Anopheles gambiae innate immune system. *PLoS Biol, 4,* e229.

Alderton LE, Spector LG, Blair CK, Roesler M, Olshan AF, et al. (2006). Child and maternal household chemical exposure and the risk of acute leukemia in children with Down's syndrome: A report from the Children's Oncology Group. *Am J Epidemiol, 164,* 212-221.

Murakami N, Xie W, Lu RC, Chen-Hwang MC, Wieraszko A, & Hwang YW. (2006). Phosphorylation of amphiphysin I by minibrain kinase/dual-specificity tyrosine phosphorylation-regulated kinase, a kinase implicated in Down syndrome. *J Biol Chem, 281,* 23712-23724.

Kubo M, & Ulrich BD. (2006). Early stage of walking: Development of control in mediolateral and anteroposterior directions. *J Mot Behav, 38,* 229-237.

Stasko MR, Scott-McKean JJ, & Costa AC. (2006). Hypothermic responses to 8-OH-DPAT in the *Ts65Dn* mouse model of Down syndrome. *Neuroreport, 17,* 837-841.

Miles S, Chapman R, & Sindberg H. (2006). Sampling context affects MLU in the language of adolescents with Down syndrome. *J Speech Lang Hear Res, 49*, 325-337.

Schrier RW. (2006). Optimal care of autosomal dominant polycystic kidney disease patients. *Nephrology (Carlton), 11*, 124-130.

Bianco K, Caughey AB, Shaffer BL, Davis R, & Norton ME. (2006). History of miscarriage and increased incidence of fetal aneuploidy in subsequent pregnancy. *Obstet Gynecol, 107*, 1098-1102.

Kuppermann M, Learman LA, Gates E, Gregorich SE, Nease RF, Jr., et al. (2006). Beyond race or ethnicity and socioeconomic status: Predictors of prenatal testing for Down syndrome. Obstet Gynecol, 107, 1087-1097.

Gropman AL, Duncan WC, & Smith AC. (2006). Neurologic and developmental features of the Smith-Magenis syndrome (del 17p11.2). *Pediatr Neurol, 34*, 337-350.

Chen MA, Lander TR, & Murphy C. (2006). Nasal health in Down syndrome: A cross-sectional study. *Otolaryngol Head Neck Surg, 134*, 741-745.

Minami T, Miura M, Aird WC, & Kodama T. (2006). Thrombin-induced auto inhibitory factor, Down syndrome critical region-1, attenuates NFAT-dependent vascular cell adhesion molecule-1 expression and inflammation in the endothelium. *J Biol Chem, 281*, 20503-20520.

Clark S, Schwalbe J, Stasko MR, Yarowsky PJ, & Costa AC. (2006). Fluoxetine rescues deficient neurogenesis in hippocampus of the *Ts65Dn* mouse model for Down syndrome. *Exp Neurol, 200*, 256-261.

Argellati F, Massone S, d'Abramo C, Marinari UM, Pronzato MA, et al. (2006). Evidence against the overexpression of *APP* in Down syndrome. *IUBMB Life, 58*, 103-106.

Abbeduto L, Murphy MM, Richmond EK, Amman A, Beth P, et al. (2006). Collaboration in referential communication: Comparison of youth with Down syndrome or fragile X syndrome. *Am J Ment Retard, 111*, 170-183.

Roper RJ, & Reeves RH. (2006). Understanding the basis for Down syndrome phenotypes. *PLoS Genet, 2*, e50.

Arron JR, Winslow MM, Polleri A, Chang CP, Wu H, et al. (2006). NFAT dysregulation by increased dosage of *DSCR1* and *DYRK1A* on chromosome 21. *Nature, 441*, 595-600.

Li CM, Guo M, Salas M, Schupf N, Silverman W, et al. (2006). Cell type-specific over-expression of chromosome 21 genes in fibroblasts and fetal hearts with trisomy 21. *BMC Med Genet, 7*, 24.

Chapman RS, Sindberg H, Bridge C, Gigstead K, & Hesketh L. (2006). Effect of memory support and elicited production on fast mapping of new words by adolescents with Down syndrome. *J Speech Lang Hear Res, 49*, 3-15.

Benson KF, & Horwitz M. (2006). Familial leukemia. *Best Pract Res Clin Haematol, 19*, 269-279.

Gardiner K. (2006). Transcriptional dysregulation in Down syndrome: predictions for altered protein complex stoichiometries and post-translational modifications, and consequences for learning/behavior genes ELK, CREB, and the estrogen and glucocorticoid receptors. *Behav Genet, 36*, 439-453.

Griffin WS. (2006). Inflammation and neurodegenerative diseases. *Am J Clin Nutr, 83*, 470S-474S.

Yoder PJ, Camarata S, Camarata M, & Williams SM. (2006). Association between differentiated processing of syllables and comprehension of grammatical morphology in children with Down syndrome. *Am J Ment Retard, 111*, 138-152.

Whitt-Glover MC, O'Neill KL, & Stettler N. (2006). Physical activity patterns in children with and without Down syndrome. *Pediatr Rehabil, 9*, 158-164.

Roper RJ, Baxter LL, Saran NG, Klinedinst DK, Beachy PA, & Reeves RH. (2006). Defective cerebellar response to mitogenic Hedgehog signaling in Down [corrected] syndrome mice. *Proc Natl Acad Sci USA, 103*, 1452-1456.

Moreira PI, Honda K, Zhu X, Nunomura A, Casadesus G, et al. (2006). Brain and brawn: Parallels in oxidative strength. *Neurology, 66*, S97-S101.

Vetrivel KS, & Thinakaran G. (2006). Amyloidogenic processing of beta-amyloid precursor protein in intracellular compartments. *Neurology, 66*, S69-S73.

Blacher J, & McIntyre LL. (2006). Syndrome specificity and behavioural disorders in young adults with intellectual disability: Cultural differences in family impact. *J Intellect Disabil Res, 50*, 184-198.

Paterson SJ, Girelli L, Butterworth B, & Karmiloff-Smith A. (2006). Are numerical impairments syndrome specific? Evidence from Williams syndrome and Down's syndrome. *J Child Psychol Psychiatry, 47*, 190-204.

Reddy UM, & Mennuti MT. (2006). Incorporating first-trimester Down syndrome studies into prenatal screening: Executive summary of the National Institute of Child Health and Human Development workshop. *Obstet Gynecol, 107*, 167-173.

Bdolah Y, Palomaki GE, Yaron Y, Bdolah-Abram T, Goldman M, et al. (2006). Circulating angiogenic proteins in trisomy 13. *Am J Obstet Gynecol, 194*, 239-245.

Dowdy-Sanders NC, & Wenger GR. (2006). Working memory in the *Ts65Dn* mouse, a model for Down syndrome. *Behav Brain Res, 168*, 349-352.

Caughey AB, Lyell DJ, Washington AE, Filly RA, & Norton ME. (2006). Ultrasound screening of fetuses at increased risk for Down syndrome: How many missed diagnoses? *Prenat Diagn, 26*, 22-27.

Lambert-Messerlian GM, Eklund EE, Malone FD, Palomaki GE, Canick JA, & D'Alton ME. (2006). Stability of first- and second-trimester serum markers after storage and shipment. *Prenat Diagn, 26*, 17-21.

Harashima C, Jacobowitz DM, Witta J, Borke RC, Best TK, et al. (2006). Abnormal expression of the G-protein-activated inwardly rectifying potassium channel 2 (GIRK2) in hippocampus, frontal cortex, and substantia nigra of *Ts65Dn* mouse: A model of Down syndrome. *J Comp Neurol, 494*, 815-833.

Kittler P, Krinsky-McHale SJ, & Devenny DA. (2006). Verbal intrusions precede memory decline in adults with Down syndrome. *J Intellect Disabil Res, 50*, 1-10.

Nelson PG, Kuddo T, Song EY, Dambrosia JM, Kohler S, et al. (2006). Selected neurotrophins, neuropeptides, and cytokines: Developmental trajectory and concentrations in neonatal blood of children with autism or Down syndrome. *Int J Dev Neurosci, 24*, 73-80.

Ge Y, Dombkowski AA, LaFiura KM, Tatman D, Yedidi RS, et al. (2006). Differential gene expression, GATA1 target genes, and the chemotherapy sensitivity of Down syndrome megakaryocytic leukemia. *Blood, 107*, 1570-1581.

Roper RJ, St. John HK, Philip J, Lawler A,& Reeves RH. (2006). Perinatal loss of *Ts65Dn* Down syndrome mice. *Genetics, 172*, 437-443.

Jenkins EC, Velinov MT, Ye L, Gu H, Li S, et al. (2006). Telomere shortening in T lymphocytes of older individuals with Down syndrome and dementia. *Neurobiol Aging, 27*, 941-945.

Kubo M, & Ulrich B. (2006). Coordination of pelvis-HAT (head, arms and trunk) in anterior-posterior and medio-lateral directions during treadmill gait in preadolescents with/without Down syndrome. *Gait Posture, 23*, 512-518.

2005

Mao R, Wang X, Spitznagel EL, Jr., Frelin LP, Ting JC, et al. (2005). Primary and secondary transcriptional effects in the developing human Down syndrome brain and heart. *Genome Biol, 6*, R107.

Brady NC, Steeples T, & Fleming K. (2005). Effects of prelinguistic communication levels on initiation and repair of communication in children with disabilities. *J Speech Lang Hear Res, 48*, 1098-1113.

Roberts J, Long SH, Malkin C, Barnes E, Skinner M, et al. (2005). A comparison of phonological skills of boys with fragile X syndrome and Down syndrome. *J Speech Lang Hear Res, 48*, 980-995.

Malone FD, Canick JA, Ball RH, Nyberg DA, Comstock CH, et al. (2005). First-trimester or second-trimester screening, or both, for Down's syndrome. *N Engl J Med, 353*, 2001-2011.

Haydar TF. (2005). Advanced microscopic imaging methods to investigate cortical development and the etiology of mental retardation. *Ment Retard Dev Disabil Res Rev, 11*, 303-316.

Sollid LM, & Lie BA. (2005). Celiac disease genetics: Current concepts and practical applications. *Clin Gastroenterol Hepatol, 3*, 843-851.

Harris CD, Ermak G, & Davies KJ. (2005). Multiple roles of the *DSCR1* (Adapt78 or RCAN1) gene and its protein product calcipressin 1 (or RCAN1) in disease. *Cell Mol Life Sci, 62*, 2477-2486.

Chang KT, & Min KT. (2005). *Drosophila melanogaster* homolog of Down syndrome critical region 1 is critical for mitochondrial function. *Nat Neurosci, 8*, 1577-1585.

Krinsky-McHale SJ, Kittler P, Brown WT, Jenkins EC, & Devenny DA. (2005). Repetition priming in adults with Williams syndrome: Age-related dissociation between implicit and explicit memory. *Am J Ment Retard, 110*, 482-496.

Kluetzman KS, Perez AV, & Crawford DR. (2005). *DSCR1* (ADAPT78) lethality: Evidence for a protective effect of trisomy 21 genes? *Biochem Biophys Res Commun, 337*, 595-601.

Sherman SL, Freeman SB, Allen EG, & Lamb NE. (2005). Risk factors for nondisjunction of trisomy 21. *Cytogenet Genome Res, 111*, 273-280.

Warburton D. (2005). Biological aging and the etiology of aneuploidy. *Cytogenet Genome Res, 111*, 266-272.

Cantor AB. (2005). GATA transcription factors in hematologic disease. *Int J Hematol, 81*, 378-384.

Cook CN, Hejna MJ, Magnuson DJ, & Lee JM. (2005). Expression of calcipressin1, an inhibitor of the phosphatase calcineurin, is altered with aging and Alzheimer's disease. *J Alzheimers Dis, 8*, 63-73.

Ravindranath Y, Chang M, Steuber CP, Becton D, Dahl G, et al. (2005). Pediatric Oncology Group (POG) studies of acute myeloid leukemia (AML): A review of four consecutive childhood AML trials conducted between 1981 and 2000. *Leukemia, 19*, 2101-2116.

Beversdorf DQ, Manning SE, Hillier A, Anderson SL, Nordgren RE, et al. (2005). Timing of prenatal stressors and autism. *J Autism Dev Disord, 35*, 471-478.

Chan B, Greenan G, McKeon F, & Ellenberger T. (2005). Identification of a peptide fragment of DSCR1 that competitively inhibits calcineurin activity *in vitro* and *in vivo*. *Proc Natl Acad Sci USA, 102*, 13075-13080.

Zigman WB, Jenkins EC, Tycko B, Schupf N, & Silverman W. (2005). Mortality is associated with apolipoprotein E epsilon4 in non-demented adults with Down syndrome. *Neurosci Lett, 390*, 93-97.

Watson FL, Puttmann-Holgado R, Thomas F, Lamar DL, Hughes M, et al. (2005). Extensive diversity of Ig-superfamily proteins in the immune system of insects. *Science, 309*, 1874-1878.

Eisenhower AS, Baker BL, & Blacher J. (2005). Preschool children with intellectual disability: Syndrome specificity, behaviour problems, and maternal well-being. *J Intellect Disabil Res, 49*, 657-671.

Fuchs KM, & Peipert JF. (2005). First trimester Down syndrome screening: Public health implications. *Semin Perinatol, 29*, 267-271.

Palomaki GE, Kloza EM, Haddow JE, Williams J, & Knight GJ. (2005). Patient and health professional acceptance of integrated serum screening for Down syndrome. *Semin Perinatol, 29*, 247-251.

Wapner RJ. (2005). First trimester screening: The BUN study. *Semin Perinatol, 29*, 236-239.

Wataganara T, Metzenbauer M, Peter I, Johnson KL, & Bianchi DW. (2005). Placental volume, as measured by 3-dimensional sonography and levels of maternal plasma cell-free fetal DNA. *Am J Obstet Gynecol, 193*, 496-500.

Tomidokoro Y, Lashley T, Rostagno A, Neubert TA, Bojsen-Moller M, et al. (2005). Familial Danish dementia: Co-existence of Danish and Alzheimer amyloid subunits (ADan AND A{beta}) in the absence of compact plaques. *J Biol Chem, 280*, 36883-36894.

Johnson MD, Yu LR, Conrads TP, Kinoshita Y, Uo T, et al. (2005). The proteomics of neurodegeneration. *Am J Pharmacogenomics, 5*, 259-270.

Akbarian S, Ruehl MG, Bliven E, Luiz LA, Peranelli AC, et al. (2005). Chromatin alterations associated with down-regulated metabolic gene expression in the prefrontal cortex of subjects with schizophrenia. *Arch Gen Psychiatry, 62*, 829-840

Pan PD, Peter I, Lambert-Messerlian GM, Canick JA, Bianchi DW, & Johnson KL. (2005). Cell-free fetal DNA levels in pregnancies conceived by IVF. *Hum Reprod, 20*, 3152-3156.

Poehlmann J, Clements M, Abbeduto L, & Farsad V. (2005). Family experiences associated with a child's diagnosis of fragile X or Down syndrome: Evidence for disruption and resilience. *Ment Retard, 43*, 255-267.

Kimura M, Cao X, Skurnick J, Cody M, Soteropoulos P, & Aviv A. (2005). Proliferation dynamics in cultured skin fibroblasts from Down syndrome subjects. *Free Radic Biol Med, 39*, 374-380.

Siarey RJ, Villar AJ, Epstein CJ, & Galdzicki Z. (2005). Abnormal synaptic plasticity in the *Ts1Cje* segmental trisomy 16 mouse model of Down syndrome. *Neuropharmacology, 49*, 122-128.

Hyman SL, & Levy SE. (2005). Introduction: Novel therapies in developmental disabilities-- hope, reason, and evidence. *Ment Retard Dev Disabil Res Rev, 11*, 107-109.

Learman LA, Drey EA, Gates EA, Kang MS, Washington AE, & Kuppermann M. (2005). Abortion attitudes of pregnant women in prenatal care. *Am J Obstet Gynecol, 192*, 1939-1945; discussion 45-47.

Birken S. (2005). Specific measurement of o-linked core 2 sugar-containing isoforms of hyperglycosylated human chorionic gonadotropin by antibody b152. *Tumour Biol, 26*, 131-141.

Dzurova D, & Pikhart H. (2005). Down syndrome, paternal age and education: Comparison of California and the Czech Republic. *BMC Public Health, 5*, 69.

Le Pecheur M, Bourdon E, Paly E, Farout L, Friguet B, & London J. (2005). Oxidized SOD1 alters proteasome activities in vitro and in the cortex of SOD1 overexpressing mice. *FEBS Lett, 579*, 3613-3618.

Ross JA, Blair CK, Olshan AF, Robison LL, Smith FO, et al. (2005). Periconceptional vitamin use and leukemia risk in children with Down syndrome: A Children's Oncology Group study. *Cancer, 104*, 405-410.

Burt DB, Primeaux-Hart S, Loveland KA, Cleveland LA, Lewis KR, et al. (2005). Aging in adults with intellectual disabilities. *Am J Ment Retard, 110*, 268-284.

Miolo G, Chapman RS, & Sindberg HA. (2005). Sentence comprehension in adolescents with Down syndrome and typically developing children: Role of sentence voice, visual context, and auditory-verbal short-term memory. *J Speech Lang Hear Res, 48*, 172-188.

Costa AC, & Grybko MJ. (2005). Deficits in hippocampal CA1 LTP induced by TBS but not HFS in the *Ts65Dn* mouse: A model of Down syndrome. *Neurosci Lett, 382*, 317-222.

Mehta PD, Patrick BA, Dalton AJ, Patel B, Mehta SP, et al. (2005). Increased serum neopterin levels in adults with Down syndrome. *J Neuroimmunol, 164*, 129-133.

Lange AW, Rothermel BA, & Yutzey KE. (2005). Restoration of *DSCR1* to disomy in the trisomy 16 mouse model of Down syndrome does not correct cardiac or craniofacial development anomalies. *Dev Dyn, 233*, 954-963.

Bahado-Singh RO, Wapner R, Thom E, Zachary J, Platt L, et al. (2005). Elevated first-trimester nuchal translucency increases the risk of congenital heart defects. *Am J Obstet Gynecol, 192,* 1357-1361.

Li Z, Godinho FJ, Klusmann JH, Garriga-Canut M, Yu C, & Orkin SH. (2005). Developmental stage-selective effect of somatically mutated leukemogenic transcription factor GATA1. *Nat Genet, 37,* 613-619.

Fidler DJ, Most DE, & Guiberson MM. (2005). Neuropsychological correlates of word identification in Down syndrome. *Res Dev Disabil, 26,* 487-501.

Muntean AG, & Crispino JD. (2005). Differential requirements for the activation domain and FOG-interaction surface of GATA-1 in megakaryocyte gene expression and development. *Blood, 106,* 1223-1231.

Levitin DJ, Cole K, Lincoln A, & Bellugi U. (2005). Aversion, awareness, and attraction: Investigating claims of hyperacusis in the Williams syndrome phenotype. *J Child Psychol Psychiatry, 46,* 514-523.

Ramakrishna N, Meeker C, Li S, Jenkins EC, Currie JR, et al. (2005). Polymerase chain reaction method to identify Down syndrome model segmentally trisomic mice. *Anal Biochem, 340,* 213-219.

Fidler DJ, Hepburn SL, Mankin G, & Rogers SJ. (2005). Praxis skills in young children with Down syndrome, other developmental disabilities, and typically developing children. *Am J Occup Ther, 59,* 129-138.

Nelson L, Johnson JK, Freedman M, Lott I, Groot J, et al. (2005). Learning and memory as a function of age in Down syndrome: A study using animal-based tasks. *Prog Neuropsychopharmacol Biol Psychiatry, 29,* 443-453.

Wilkinson KM. (2005). Disambiguation and mapping of new word meanings by individuals with intellectual/developmental disabilities. *Am J Ment Retard, 110,* 71-86.

Capone GT, Grados MA, Kaufmann WE, Bernad-Ripoll S, & Jewell A. (2005). Down syndrome and comorbid autism-spectrum disorder: Characterization using the aberrant behavior checklist. *Am J Med Genet A, 134,* 373-380.

Helguera P, Pelsman A, Pigino G, Wolvetang E, Head E, & Busciglio J. (2005). ets-2 promotes the activation of a mitochondrial death pathway in Down's syndrome neurons. *J Neurosci, 25,* 2295-2303.

Haacke EM, Cheng NY, House MJ, Liu Q, Neelavalli J, et al. (2005). Imaging iron stores in the brain using magnetic resonance imaging. *Magn Reson Imaging, 23,* 1-25.

Caughey AB. (2005). Cost-effectiveness analysis of prenatal diagnosis: Methodological issues and concerns. *Gynecol Obstet Invest, 60,* 11-18.

Crispino JD. (2005). GATA1 in normal and malignant hematopoiesis. *Semin Cell Dev Biol, 16*, 137-147.

Dauphinot L, Lyle R, Rivals I, Dang MT, Moldrich RX, et al. (2005). The cerebellar transcriptome during postnatal development of the *Ts1Cje* mouse, a segmental trisomy model for Down syndrome. *Hum Mol Genet, 14*, 373-384.

Tseng BP, Kitazawa M, & LaFerla FM. (2004). Amyloid beta-peptide: The inside story. *Curr Alzheimer Res, 1*, 231-239.

Bird EK, Chapman RS, & Schwartz SE. (2004). Fast mapping of words and story recall by individuals with Down syndrome. *J Speech Lang Hear Res, 47*, 1286-1300.

Levitin DJ, Cole K, Chiles M, Lai Z, Lincoln A, & Bellugi U. (2004). Characterizing the musical phenotype in individuals with Williams syndrome. *Child Neuropsychol, 10*, 223-247.

FIGURE 1: JOURNAL PUBLICATIONS RELATED TO DOWN SYNDROME THAT RESULTED FROM NIH SUPPORT

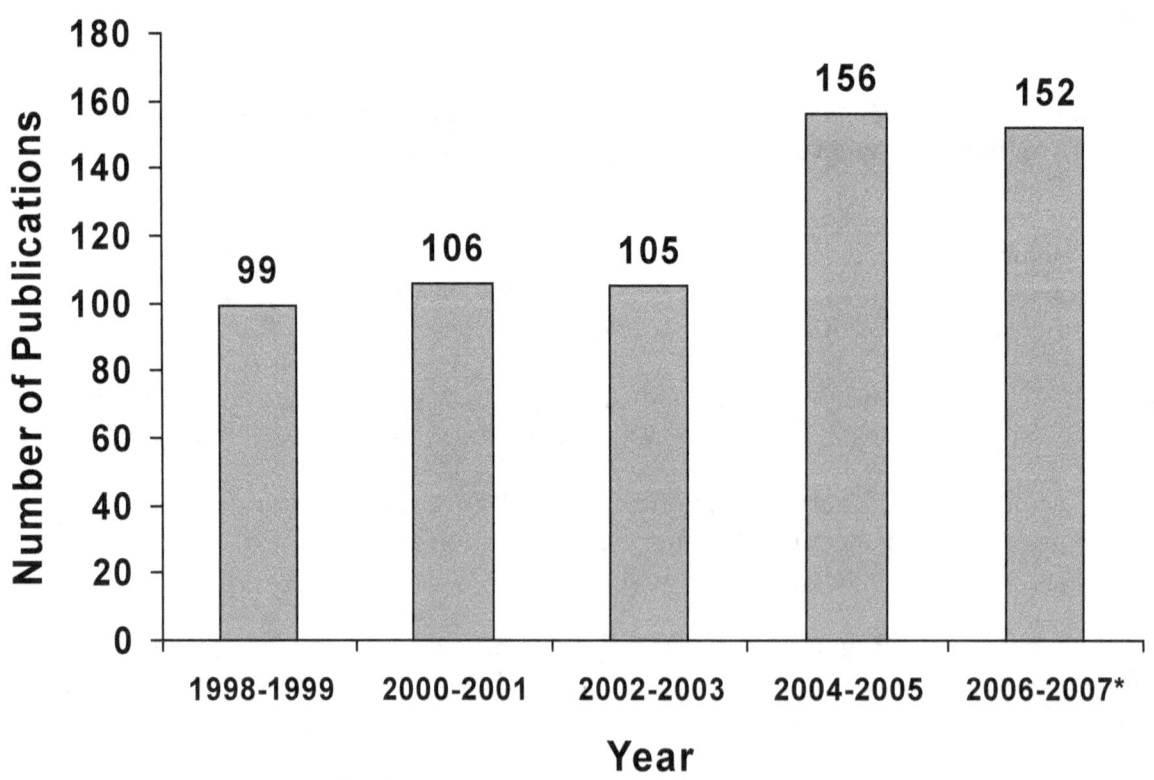

* Estimated